The Senior Fitness Blueprint

Creating a Customized Fitness Strategy to Enhance Strength, Balance, and Coordination with SIMPLE Chair Exercises

Mel Don, PT

CONTENTS

Introduction ... 1

1. Foundations of Balance and Coordination ... 5

2. Safety and Injury Prevention ... 19

3. Progressive Balance Exercises ... 39

4. Holistic Health and Mindfulness ... 49

5. Addressing Common Physical Limitations ... 61

6. Motivational Strategies and Long-term Habits ... 73

7. Exercises for Everyday Independence ... 83

8. Advanced Techniques for Improved Stability ... 93

Conclusion ... 112

Appendix ... 115

References ... 127

INTRODUCTION

My Grandma visiting me at my place of work DNA FITNESS
Montreal

Growing up on a rural farm, under the nurturing guidance of my grandmother, has filled my life with many treasured memories. These experiences have deeply influenced who I am today. I vividly recall sitting on a worn-out bucket amid her vibrant garden, the taste of fresh tomatoes bursting with flavor as we shared those quiet moments. She taught me the gentle art of feeding baby goats, a task that required patience and a soft touch, lessons that have stayed with me throughout my life. Our walks in the forest during the brisk Canadian winters, collecting maple syrup, were magical adventures, transforming the cold into a sweet wonderland. These experiences, rich in simplicity and love, shaped my appreciation for life's simple joys and the importance of maintaining a healthy, active lifestyle.

My grandmother, who celebrated her 95th birthday as I pen these words, epitomizes strength and resilience. Her journey through life has been anything but easy. Born in Italy during World War II, she encountered obstacles that tested her will. Despite wartime adversities, she never allowed her circumstances to define her future. In the years following the war, she boldly decided to immigrate to Canada. This move demanded learning a new language and adapting to a different culture while embracing her role as a new mother. Her ability to navigate these monumental changes, find work, and build a life in a foreign land exemplifies the resilience that has characterized her ever since. Watching her gracefully navigate her later years—continually staying active through walking, singing, dancing, and exercising—only deepened my respect and admiration for her. It was this unwavering spirit and her ability to maintain balance, both literally and figuratively, through the ebbs and flows of life, that inspired me to create this book. Her life was a testament to the importance of cultivating strength and balance as we age, demonstrating that independence is not just a state of being but a skill that can be honed with the right mindset and tools.

My journey to this point has been anything but straightforward. I spent a decade as a gymnast, pushing my body to its limits. The injuries were part of the package. Navigating through knee and ankle injuries tested my determination deeply. It was only later that I discovered my back had also suffered, leading to a diagnosis of severe degenerative disk disease in my lower spine—a consequence of the relentless impact of my athletic pursuits. As is often the case for former athletes, the initial post-retirement years were physically and mentally demanding. The absence of a structured routine and clear goals led to a decline into an unhealthy lifestyle, which was accompanied by significant weight gain, illness, and depression. After being diagnosed with rheumatoid arthritis in 2005, I decided that enough was enough and went on to pursue a happier life by exercising and adopting healthier eating habits. My life now is one of health and joy, surrounded by my loving husband and two wonderful kids.

At this pivotal moment in my journey, fate introduced me to my future husband, a fellow personal trainer who founded DNA FITNESS in Montreal, Canada. Joining the DNA team transformed my life, deepening my passion for fitness and broadening my expertise. I earned certifications in personal training, yoga, prenatal yoga, and prenatal strength training, and it was at this point that I dove into senior fitness training.

Over the past 14 years, I've been incredibly fortunate to guide and support numerous senior clients on their fitness journeys. Witnessing their unwavering determination and indomitable spirit firsthand has not only inspired me but also deepened my commitment to creating accessible fitness solutions for seniors. Their perseverance and zest for life remind me every day why I chose this path.

The primary purpose of this book is simple. I intend to significantly improve your quality of life by guiding you toward a healthier and more mobile lifestyle, with a focus on bolstering your balance and coordination. It has been meticulously crafted to empower you with independence and reinforce your confidence in everyday activities. You are deserving of a life where movement is effortless and your body feels robust.

What sets this book apart is the blend of expertise and personal experience from clients of all age levels and mobility. My background as a gymnast and personal trainer informs every exercise. You won't need special equipment. Just a chair and some space to move. This holistic approach makes the program accessible to everyone at any age.

This book is meticulously structured to equip you with the tools and the wisdom gleaned from my past experiences with my senior clients, guiding you confidently into this transformative journey. It delves into the nuances of navigating physical limitations caused by various illnesses, offering thoughtful modifications to tailor each exercise to your unique needs. It provides valuable tips on injury prevention, mindfulness, and nutrition because true health involves the mind and body working in harmony. Each exercise can be adapted to suit your individual needs, making the program truly yours.

To enhance your exercise experience and offer you complimentary resources for your fitness journey, this book features QR codes. These distinct square barcodes can be easily scanned using your smartphone or tablet, leading you directly to a webpage or resource designed to support you in achieving your fitness objectives. To use the QR codes, follow these steps:

1. **Use Your Smartphone or Tablet**: Make sure you have a device with a camera.

2. **Open Your Camera App**: Most smartphones have a built-in camera that can scan QR codes. To use it, launch the Camera as if you're taking a picture.

3. **Aim the Camera at the QR Code**: Hold your phone or tablet steady and point the Camera at the QR code in the book. Ensure the code is well-lit and clear.

4. **Tap the Notification**: A notification should pop up on your screen after a few moments. Tap it to access the content linked to the QR code.

As you begin this journey, know that I understand the challenges you face. Throughout my career, I've witnessed incredible transformations among my cherished clients, whose fitness levels varied widely—from clients who use wheelchairs to those grappling with severe arthritis and osteoporosis; every person has witnessed enhancements in their overall fitness and self-confidence. This book is crafted as a tool, designed with compassion and understanding, aiming to significantly enhance your quality of life. Together, we can work towards a better you. Let's begin.

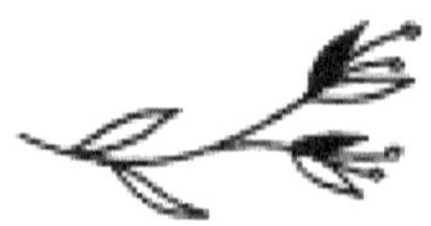

1

——— ◆ ———

Foundations of Balance and Coordination

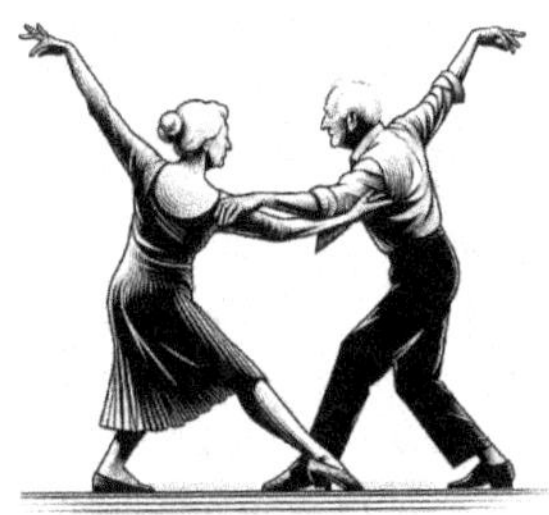 My grandmother, an embodiment of unwavering resilience, navigates her golden years with a steadiness that, to this day, captives me. Her movements, whether she's preparing those delicious home-cooked Italian meals from scratch or taking leisurely walks with me through the neighbourhood, serve as a living testament to her exceptional mastery of strength, balance, and coordination.

Understanding Balance and Coordination

Balance and coordination are crucial in our daily lives and are especially vital for seniors. As we grow older, our bodies experience inevitable changes that impact our strength, balance, and coordination. Acknowledging the harsh reality that falls have become our senior community's leading cause of injury is crucial. Yet, there's an encouraging aspect to this: these accidents are largely preventable. By improving your balance, coordination, and overall strength, you can reduce your fall risk and enhance your ability to perform everyday activities confidently and easily.

Our bodies have intricate systems designed to maintain balance. At the center of these systems is the vestibular apparatus, nestled within the inner ear. This system is crucial for keeping our equilibrium and understanding where we are in space. For example, when we turn our heads, the vestibular system allows us to adjust without losing our balance. Another essential element is proprioception, our innate sense of body position. Thanks to proprioception, we can perform tasks like reaching for a glass without needing to watch our hands closely. These, along with our senses of sight and touch, form a sophisticated balance mechanism that helps us navigate the world smoothly and efficiently.

Research demonstrates that participating in targeted exercises, which we will introduce in the following sections, can substantially enhance stability and coordination for individuals of all ages. By dedicating time to regular practice, you can fortify the underlying systems responsible for these crucial functions. This improvement empowers you to navigate your daily activities with increased confidence and independence, contributing to a more active and fulfilling lifestyle.

In the coming pages, we'll explore practical and enjoyable exercises to build physical strength geared toward independence and well-being. This journey is yours to take, and I'm here to guide you every step of the way!

The Role of Balance in Daily Activities

The act of standing up from a chair requires more balance than one might initially think. As you transition from sitting to standing, your body must shift its center of gravity, engage muscles in the legs and core, and stabilize to avoid toppling over. This is balance in action. Reaching for an item on a high shelf is another daily task that calls for balance. You extend your arm while your body works to keep you stable. These are just a few simple examples of how balance is woven into the fabric of our everyday lives.

Maintaining balance is crucial for independence. It allows you to carry out household chores without needing assistance, giving you the freedom to move about your home confidently. When balance is compromised, even simple tasks can become daunting obstacles. Good balance provides the confidence to navigate social settings and enjoy outdoor activities, which can positively impact your mental well-being. We will incorporate exercises that mimic everyday movements to integrate balance more seamlessly into daily life.

The heel-to-toe walk, for instance, is a simple exercise that can be performed anywhere.

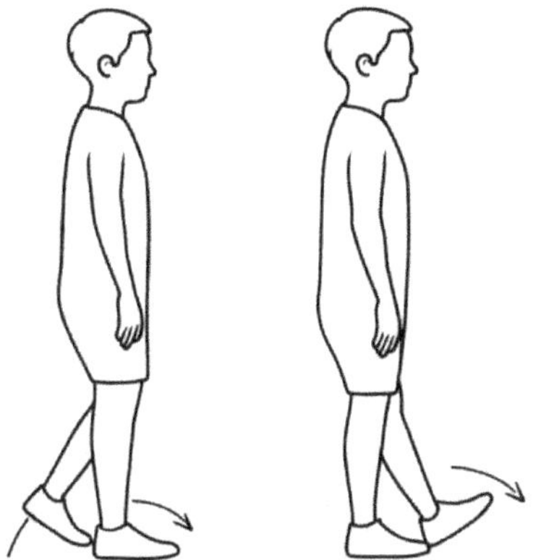

By walking in a straight line and placing one foot directly in front of the other as if on a tightrope, you engage the same muscles and balance systems used in walking up stairs or navigating narrow spaces.

Another example of an exercise that offers practical balance is the single-leg stand. To perform this exercise, stand on one leg while holding onto a stable chair or surface for support, gradually building the ability to maintain balance without assistance.

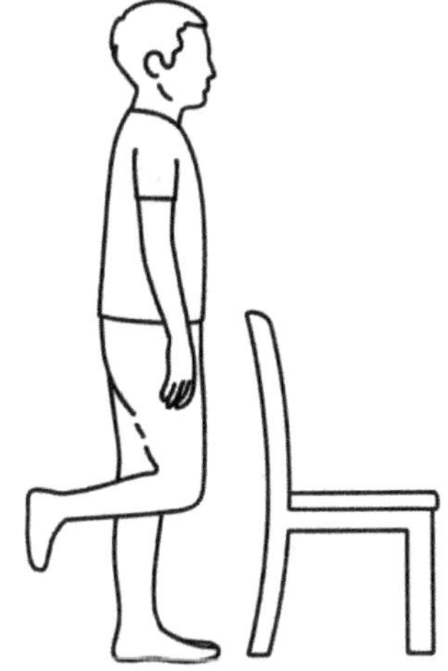

These exercises improve physical stability and increase confidence in performing daily tasks. Incorporating these exercises into your routine reinforces the balance required for everyday activities. It's about making small, consistent efforts that enhance balance over time. With improved balance, tasks that once seemed daunting become more manageable, and activities that were once avoided can now be approached enthusiastically. Balance is not just a skill; it's a key to unlocking a more independent and fulfilling life.

How Coordination Affects Mobility

Coordination plays a pivotal role in how we move, influencing our ability to navigate the world easily, such as walking down a sidewalk. Many of us do it without a second thought, yet it requires coordination between the arms and legs. As one foot steps forward, the opposite arm swings to maintain balance and keep us steady. This coordination becomes even more crucial as we age, when our bodies might not respond as they once did.

Similarly, hand-eye coordination is vital for tasks that involve reaching and grasping. Picture yourself reaching for a book on a shelf. Your eyes gauge the distance, your brain calculates the reach, and your hand moves to grasp the object. This is coordination at work, allowing you to interact with your environment smoothly. It's a skill we often take for granted, but its importance becomes apparent when it begins to falter. Without effective coordination, even the simplest of tasks can become challenging, impacting our overall mobility and independence.

A simple ball toss with alternating hands can help improve coordination. This activity engages hand-eye coordination and requires mental focus, enhancing your ability to multitask. Cross-body movement, such as touching your right hand to your left knee, is another example of an exercise that can challenge your coordination further. These exercises connect the brain's hemispheres, boosting overall coordination and mobility.

Some benefits of enhanced coordination, which extend beyond physical movement, are how it contributes to better cardiovascular fitness. Any activity that involves coordination often elevates heart rate and boosts cardiovascular health. Improved coordination also supports joint health and flexibility since you engage different muscles and joints. On the plus side, this does help reduce the risk of injury and maintain flexibility.

Identifying Balance Challenges in Seniors

As we age, our bodies undergo various changes that can impact balance. One of the most common issues faced by seniors is vertigo—a sensation of spinning or dizziness that can strike unexpectedly. It's often linked to inner ear problems, but sometimes the cause remains elusive, leaving individuals feeling disoriented and unsteady. This can be especially troubling when standing up quickly or turning suddenly. Additionally, certain medical conditions such as arthritis, osteoporosis, and muscle weakness emerge as a significant challenge among seniors. Over time, muscles naturally diminish in mass and strength, undermining stability and heightening the risk of falls. This muscle decline can make activities that once seemed simple, like rising from a chair or crossing a room, become more intimidating. Recognizing these challenges is the first step in addressing them effectively.

In the Appendix, you will find a home self-assessment document, catering to both seated and standing mobility, designed to help you monitor and celebrate your progress. I would suggest to retest every 6 to 8 weeks to start seeing a nice progression.

Essential Equipment-Free Exercises

In the world of fitness, equipment can often seem like a barrier. It can be costly, cumbersome, and sometimes downright intimidating. For seniors, the appeal of equipment-free exercises lies in their simplicity and accessibility. You don't need a gym membership or fancy machines to improve your health. These exercises can be performed in the comfort of your home.

Additionally, these exercises offer an economic advantage. They eliminate the need for expensive gear, making fitness accessible to anyone willing to engage. The beauty of this approach is that it empowers you to maintain your health on your terms, wherever you feel most comfortable.

Now, let's explore core exercises that lay the foundation for improved balance and coordination, beginning with chair squats.

This exercise engages the muscles in your legs and core, which are essential for stability. Stand in front of a sturdy chair, your feet hip-width apart, and gently lower yourself as if to sit down, stopping just above the seat. Keep your back straight and your eyes forward. Engage your core. To do this, envision yourself pulling your belly button towards your spine. Once you have engaged your core, rise back to standing. Repeat this movement with a particular focus on 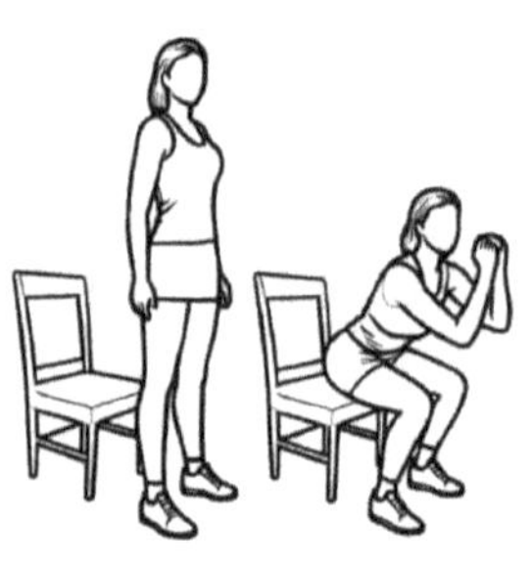 form. Finally, a mistake I often need to correct with my clients is ensuring they keep their knees from extending beyond their toes; this common mistake can stress your joints.

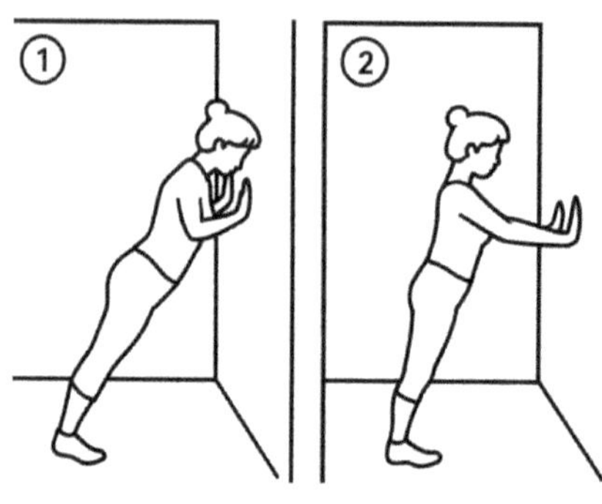

Wall push-ups offer another excellent no-equipment option. Stand facing a wall, arms extended at shoulder height, hands flat against the surface. Step back slightly and lean into the wall, bending your elbows to lower your body, then push back to the starting position. This exercise strengthens your upper body and core while maintaining balance.

These foundational exercises can be adjusted to suit various fitness levels. If standing is challenging, try seated versions. For chair squats, sit and stand from the chair, using your arms for support if needed. This modification allows you to build strength gradually. For those seeking more challenge, increase the repetitions or hold the squat position longer to intensify the workout. Wall push-ups can also be made more demanding by stepping further from the wall or performing them on a lower surface like a countertop.

The key is to ensure that each movement is deliberate and controlled, focusing on quality over quantity. Ensuring safety through meticulous attention to detail is paramount when performing these exercises. Begin every session with a thorough warm-up to prepare your body for the workout ahead.

A simple yet effective warm-up could include gentle marching on the spot for those able to stand or a seated march for those who prefer or require a chair-based exercise.

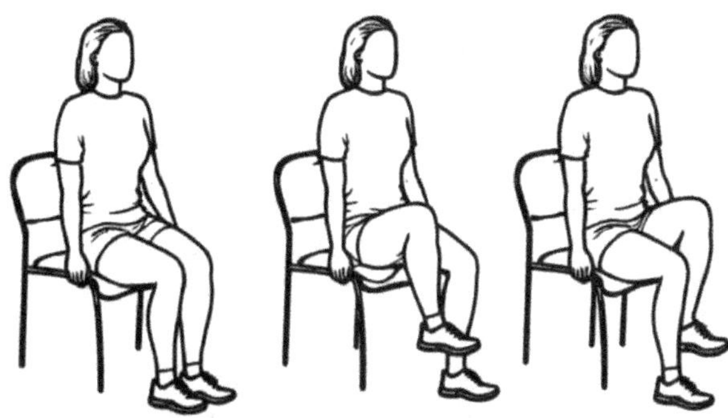

Enhance this warm-up by incorporating arm circles. Slowly rotate your arms in a controlled manner to loosen the shoulder joints and increase blood flow to your muscles.

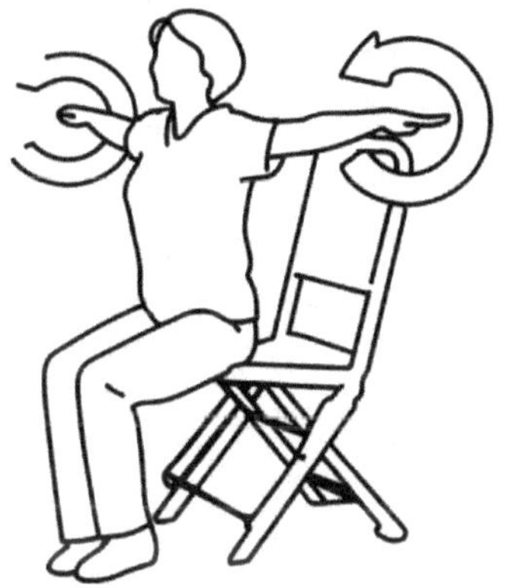

As you transition into the main exercises, it's crucial to maintain proper posture. This involves standing or sitting straight, shoulders back, and engaging your core muscles to support your spine.

Equally important is the rhythm of your breathing; strive to inhale deeply through your nose and exhale slowly through your mouth. This controlled breathing oxygenates your muscles and promotes relaxation and focus, enabling you to perform each exercise with greater precision. Listening to your body's signals is another key aspect of safely executing these exercises. If you experience any discomfort, it's advisable to pause and rest. Pushing through pain could lead to injury, which is counterproductive to your goal of strengthening and stabilizing your body. Remember, the objective here is not to rush through the routines or strain beyond your limits but to gradually build your physical capabilities. Adopting these exercises into your daily routine offers more than just physical health benefits; it lays the foundation for a lifestyle characterized by greater independence and overall well-being. Focusing on technique, posture, and proper breathing ensures a safe and effective workout supporting your journey toward a more active and fulfilling life.

Setting Personal Fitness Goals

Setting personal fitness goals is a crucial first step that adds direction and purpose to your fitness journey, turning vague wishes into actionable plans. To make these goals achievable and practical, they must be carefully tailored to be realistic and attainable. This is where the SMART framework can guide you. It outlines how to craft goals that are Specific, pinpointing precisely what you aim to accomplish; Measurable, so you can track your progress and recognize when you've achieved your goals; Achievable, to ensure your goals are within your reach given your current abilities and resources; Relevant, so they align with your personal values and broader life goals; and Time-bound, with a clear deadline to keep you focused and motivated. By adopting this structured approach, you're not just daydreaming about better health and wellness but setting yourself up for tangible success on your journey toward enhanced fitness.

Breaking down the SMART framework further, we find that a specific goal avoids vagueness and defines clear parameters for success. For example, choosing to embark on a 20-minute walk every morning is significantly more directive and manageable than a broad desire to "exercise more." This specificity narrows focus and simplifies decision-making.

A goal must have quantifiable indicators of progress to be measurable. This could mean tracking the number of steps walked each day with a pedometer or noting the minutes spent actively engaging in physical activity. Such metrics allow for tangible benchmarks of achievement, offering concrete evidence of your journey toward your fitness aspirations.

An achievable goal considers your current physical condition, health status, and lifestyle. It challenges you without pushing beyond your limits, ensuring that the objectives set are within your grasp. This element of the framework encourages a realistic assessment of what you can accomplish, fostering progress while avoiding discouragement.

Relevance ensures that your fitness goals align with your values, interests, and broader objectives. A goal that matters deeply to you is inherently more motivating. If enhancing your garden's beauty through regular upkeep is important, setting a fitness goal around gardening activities can imbue your physical efforts with a sense of purpose and joy.

Lastly, time-bound goals are those with a set deadline. This could range from short-term goals, like improving balance within a month, to long-term ambitions, such as participating in a community walkathon six months down the line. Deadlines introduce a sense of urgency and commitment, compelling action, and focus on achieving timely accomplishment.

By carefully incorporating the SMART criteria into your fitness objectives, you establish a tailored and achievable plan for success. This method provides clear guidance and infuses your fitness journey with purpose, motivation, and a deep sense of personal relevance.

Personalization is crucial when it comes to goal-setting, especially in fitness. Each person's body and circumstances are unique, so it's essential to tailor goals to fit your needs and abilities. Consider your health conditions—perhaps you've been managing arthritis or recovering from surgery. These factors should influence your goals, ensuring they are both challenging and considerate of your health. Incorporate your interests and preferences into your goals, too. If you enjoy gardening, set a goal to spend more time tending to your plants to stay active. This approach makes goals more enjoyable and will help increase the likelihood of sticking to them.

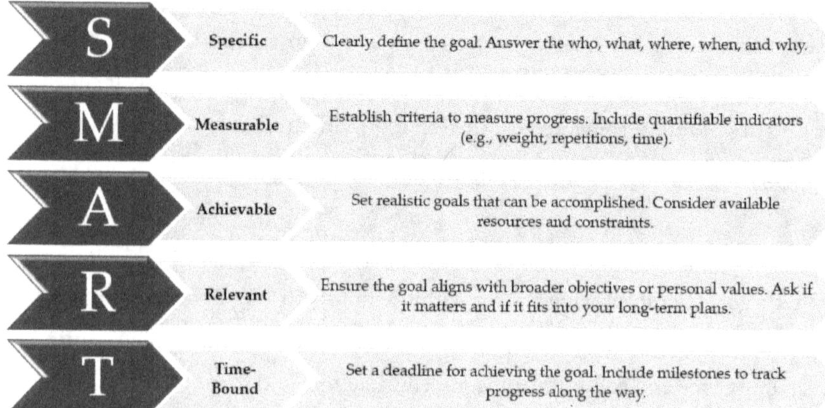

Below you will find a tool I created to help you set your SMART Goals.

Another significant challenge is maintaining motivation, particularly when focusing on enhancing balance and coordination. The use of a fitness journal , as a part of your daily routine is an incredibly effective way to strengthen your dedication. It is more than simply logging exercises. It involves documenting your personal journey, capturing the **subtle improvements** in your balance and coordination, and learning how your body adapts and strengthens over time. By reflecting on these entries, you can visually track your progress, identify patterns, and celebrate the milestones of your journey towards greater stability and independence. Documenting your journey in a journal becomes a profound source of motivation, offering a vivid, tangible representation of your progress.

This practice highlights the fact that every single effort, regardless of its perceived size, acts as a crucial step forward in your journey to enhanced balance, coordination, and overall well-being. Celebrating these milestones is vital. They are not just achievements but **pivotal moments** of transformation. These celebrations are vital. They reinforce positive behaviors, uplift your spirit, and remind you why you started. In light of this, I've crafted an Exercise Log designed to complement your journey. This log isn't just a tool for tracking; it's a companion on your path to a more balanced, coordinated, and fulfilling life. You'll have the capability to monitor not just your exercises but also various factors that influence your body, including the weather, your mood, water consumption, daily meals, and step count, while also maintaining a journal for notes.

You can download the Planner using this QR code. A quick view of what it resembles is on the following page.

Todays Plan

M T W T F S S   Date:

Weather

Mood

Exercise	Rep	Set

Notes

Top 3 Priorities

1.
2.
3.

To-Do List

○
○
○
○
○
○

Breakfast

Lunch

Dinner

Snacks

Water Today

Steps Today

Incorporating a support system into your fitness regimen can profoundly enhance your journey toward better balance and coordination. Encourage family and friends to join you in your exercises, transforming your workout sessions into shared, joyous experiences.

Imagine starting your day with a refreshing morning walk accompanied by a neighbour or sharing a laughter-filled exercise session with your partner right in your living room. These moments of togetherness fortify your relationships and ensure a layer of accountability, making it more likely for you to stick with your routine. Setting personal fitness goals transcends the realm of mere physical transformation. It's about adopting a growth mindset that positions you as the captain of your health and well-being. Each goal you set and achieve not only bolsters your confidence in your physical capabilities but also in your ability to surmount life's hurdles. As you advance through your strength, balance and coordination program, you'll come to see these goals as more than just milestones; they are the beacons leading you toward a life brimming with activity and vitality. By thoughtfully setting and pursuing these objectives, you unlock a universe of potential, demonstrating with each step that your strength and resolve are the cornerstones of a fulfilling, vibrant life.

2

SAFETY AND INJURY PREVENTION

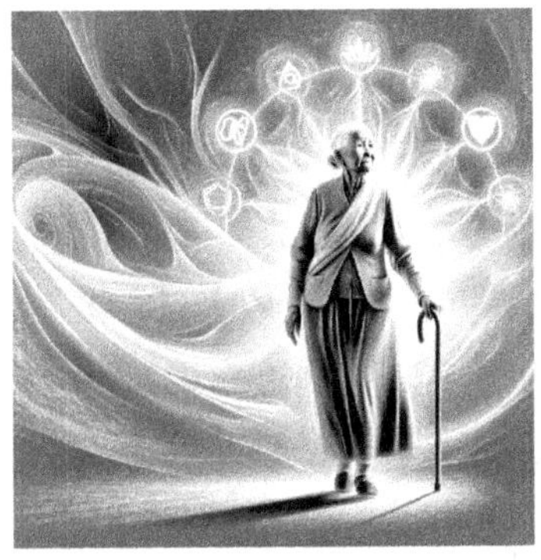

Before diving into an exercise routine, one crucial step can make all the difference in how you feel during and after your workout: the warm-up. Think of it as a welcoming ritual for your body, a gentle nudge to awaken your muscles and joints, preparing them for the activity ahead. This simple yet powerful start can be your most helpful ally in preventing injuries and maximizing the benefits of your exercises.

Warming up is a preliminary step and a cornerstone of safe and effective exercise, particularly for older adults. Our bodies can become more susceptible to strains and injuries as we age. A proper warm-up increases blood flow to your muscles, like delivering a fresh fuel supply to an engine, making your body more efficient and resilient. Enhanced joint flexibility is another key benefit. As your joints receive more circulation, they become more pliable, allowing you to move with greater ease and less risk of strain. This preparation is essential, enabling you to confidently engage in your exercises and reduce the likelihood of discomfort or injury.

The duration and intensity of your warm-up are just as important as the exercises themselves. Aim for a warm-up that lasts between five to ten minutes. This timeframe allows your body to gradually transition from a state of rest to one of activity. Start slowly, focusing on the quality of your movements rather than speed. You can gently increase the intensity as your muscles begin to warm, but remember to listen to your body and adjust as needed. The goal is to feel invigorated, not exhausted, as you move into your exercise routine.

A widespread misconception suggests that only high-intensity workouts require warm-ups. This belief is unfounded and overlooks the universal benefits of warming up. Warm-up exercises are essential, irrespective of the workout's intensity. They ready your body for a range of activities, from a gentle walk to a vigorous strength-training session. Including a warm-up in your exercise regimen is a proactive step toward safeguarding your health and maximizing the effectiveness of your workout.

Preventive Measures to Prevent Falls

Several everyday scenarios can lead to falls. Recognizing these hazards is crucial in fall prevention. By being aware of these risks, you can take proactive steps, implementing simple yet impactful modifications that significantly diminish the chances of a fall. For example, installing grab bars can be a game changer. These provide sturdy support, allowing you to maneuver confidently, whether stepping in or out of the shower or using the toilet. Similarly, ensuring adequate lighting in hallways and staircases can make a difference. Shadows and poor visibility can obscure obstacles, increasing the risk of a misstep. Bright, clear lighting helps you see clearly, enabling safer navigation through your home. Consider adding nightlights to guide your path during those late-night trips. These modifications are small investments that yield big returns in safety and peace of mind.

In training, the importance of appropriate footwear cannot be overstressed. Your shoes act as foundational support, playing a pivotal role in maintaining stability and preventing slips, which are common causes for concern among seniors. The right pair of non-slip shoes with substantial support can be one of the best methods to prevent falls. When selecting footwear, prioritize shoes with a firm grip on the sole, ensuring a secure footing on various surfaces. A snug fit is equally important, as it supports your arches, reducing the risk of foot fatigue and missteps.

Additionally, opt for shoes designed with adequate cushioning, as they offer better shock absorption, contributing to overall joint health. Avoid wearing slippers or footwear with smooth soles indoors, as these can significantly increase the risk of slips and falls, especially on slick surfaces like tile or hardwood floors. Instead, choose shoes that securely fasten to your feet and feature a textured sole for enhanced grip. This careful selection of footwear is not merely a precaution but a crucial investment in your daily safety and mobility. Choosing shoes that ensure stability and comfort empowers you to move confidently and freely, making each step secure. It is a simple yet effective measure in avoiding unnecessary injury and help prevent falls, ensuring that you can engage in daily activities and exercises with assurance and ease.

Safe Exercise Practices at Home

Creating a safe exercise environment at home is essential in ensuring a rewarding workout experience, especially as we age. The first thing to consider is your workout space. It should be free of clutter and obstacles. Imagine moving through your home with the same freedom you would feel in a wide-open field. That sense of freedom starts with eliminating tripping hazards like loose rugs, scattered shoes, or even electrical cords that might cross your path.

Ensuring the stability of any furniture you employ for support during your exercises is crucial for maintaining a safe workout environment at home. Whether utilizing a chair for seated exercises or a table to aid in balance activities, it is imperative that these items are robust enough to bear your weight securely. The last thing you want is for your support to wobble or shift unpredictably as you lean or hold onto it during your exercise routines.

To enhance the safety and stability of these supports, consider affixing furniture pads or anti-slip grips underneath their legs. These simple additions can significantly reduce the risk of the furniture slipping or moving out of place, providing a solid and dependable base for your exercises. This added stability serves as a safety net, offering you peace of mind and allowing you to concentrate fully on your exercises. With these precautions in place, you can trust in the reliability of your surroundings and dedicate your full attention to executing your movements with precision and care, secure in the knowledge that your chosen supports will steadfastly assist you throughout your workout session.

Body awareness is a crucial component of safe exercise, often overlooked but incredibly powerful. It involves being mindful of how your body moves and feels during your workout. Slow and controlled movements are key. Picture yourself moving through a series of gentle stretches, feeling each muscle elongate and contract. This mindfulness reduces the risk of injury by allowing you to notice any tension or discomfort before it becomes problematic. Maintain proper posture throughout, keeping your spine aligned and your core engaged. This conscious attention to your body's position helps prevent strain and enhances the effectiveness of your exercises.

Before you begin any exercise routine, take a moment to conduct a few safety checks. Ensure that any equipment you plan to use is stable and in good condition. A quick inspection can save you from potential mishaps. Additionally, confirm that you have sufficient space to move freely. This is particularly important if you're trying new exercises that might require more room than usual. Once you've ensured your space is secure, you can exercise with peace of mind, knowing that you've minimized the risk of injury.

Proper hydration and ventilation are critical yet frequently undervalued components of exercise safety. They warrant as much attention as the physical activities themselves. Ensuring you have a water bottle within easy reach during your workouts is essential. Dehydration can sneak up, particularly in seniors, leading to symptoms like fatigue, dizziness, and confusion, which can significantly detract from the effectiveness and safety of your exercise routine. Regular sips of water help maintain hydration levels, support your body's functions and enhance endurance, allowing you to complete your workouts without unnecessary discomfort. Equally important is the quality of the air in your workout space. A well-ventilated area ensures that fresh air continuously circulates, replacing any stale or oxygen-depleted air. This is particularly crucial when exercising indoors, where limited airflow can lead to a buildup of carbon dioxide, making breathing more laborious and potentially diminishing your performance. Opening windows or using fans can aid in maintaining a flow of fresh air, thereby keeping the environment comfortable and conducive to exertion. Moreover, proper ventilation helps regulate temperature, preventing your workout space from becoming excessively warm. A cooler environment not only makes for a more pleasant exercise experience but also helps prevent overheating, which can lead to heat exhaustion, a condition particularly risky for seniors. By integrating these practices into your routine, your home transforms into a sanctuary for safe and effective exercise. This not only empowers you to engage in your fitness journey with greater confidence but also enhances your overall well-being, allowing you to reap the full benefits of your exercise regimen.

Safety Checklist for Home Workouts

- **Clear Space:** Remove obstacles and clutter.

- **Stable** Support: Ensure furniture is sturdy.

- **Body Awareness**: Focus on posture and controlled movements.

- **Safety Checks**: Verify equipment stability and space.

- **Hydration:** Keep water handy for your exercise session.

- **Ventilation:** Ensure the room is well-ventilated for comfort.

Recognizing and Addressing Pain

Grasping the subtleties of pain is critical, particularly when engaging in physical activities. It's essential to understand that not all pain experienced during or after exercise is cause for alarm; in fact, some discomfort can serve as a marker of progress, while other types might indicate potential injury or overexertion. One common form of discomfort is muscle soreness, which many interpret as a hallmark of an effective workout. This type of soreness, characterized by a dull and aching sensation, is a direct result of your muscles responding to the physical demands placed upon them. Typically, this sensation emerges after trying new exercises or increasing the intensity of your workouts and generally subsides within a few days. Often termed "good pain," this soreness signifies that your muscles are undergoing adaptation processes, becoming stronger and more resilient as a result of the workout's challenges.

Conversely, experiencing sharp, localized joint pain serves as a critical warning signal. This type of discomfort, marked by its intensity and precise location, often suggests an underlying issue that requires immediate attention. Ignoring such pain increases the risk of exacerbating potential injuries or strains, which could significantly hinder your mobility and overall well-being. In addition to sharp pain, the presence of inflammation in a joint—evidenced by symptoms such as swelling, redness, or a sensation of warmth—demands careful consideration. These inflammatory markers are your body's method of indicating that something is amiss, prompting you to temporarily halt your activities to evaluate your condition. Neglecting these signs not only prolongs recovery but may also lead to more severe complications. It is crucial, therefore, to listen to your body's signals, distinguishing between normal exercise-induced discomfort and indicators of potential harm. This discernment allows you to make informed decisions about your exercise regimen, ensuring your continued health and mobility.

As you engage in exercises, you might encounter common discomforts. Muscle cramps are sudden, involuntary contractions that can be pretty painful. They often occur when a muscle is overworked or dehydrated. Joint discomfort, another common issue, might arise from repetitive movements or incorrect form. It's important to differentiate between temporary discomfort and ongoing pain that might indicate a more serious problem. Recognizing these sensations allows you to address them promptly, preventing further complications.

There are several strategies to manage pain effectively during and after exercise. Applying ice can reduce inflammation and numb sharp pain, while heat packs can relax tight muscles and improve blood flow.

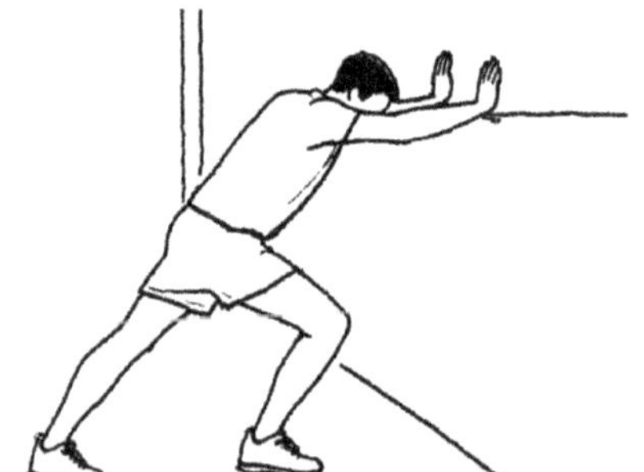

Gentle stretching is another valuable tool. It helps to relieve tension and maintain flexibility. For instance, if your calves feel tight, a simple calf stretch against the wall can provide relief.

Incorporating rest days into your routine is also beneficial, allowing your body time to recover and heal. Rest doesn't mean inactivity; it's simply a chance to engage in low-impact activities like walking or yoga, which keep you moving without overstraining your muscles.

If pain persists I suggest to consult with healthcare professional to address the issue right away. Too many times we tend to try to push through the pain. You do not want to develop a chronic condition. Regular check-ups with your doctor can provide insights into your overall health and guide you on the best practices for exercise. They can help identify underlying issues that might be contributing to your discomfort. Addressing pain promptly and effectively not only enhances your physical health but also boosts your confidence in maintaining an active lifestyle.

Modifying Exercises for Health Conditions

The principle of individualized exercise programming is paramount, mainly when designing routines for seniors. Recognizing the diverse spectrum of physical capabilities among older adults is essential. My experience with senior clients has spanned a broad range of mobility levels, from those who can engage in weightlifting to individuals who navigate their daily lives from a wheelchair. Despite these differences in mobility, it's crucial to understand that effective and comprehensive workouts are achievable for all. For my clients who use wheelchairs, we've successfully adapted exercises to ensure that they can still target and strengthen all major muscle groups. This adaptability underscores the importance of tailoring exercise routines to meet each individual's specific health and mobility needs, ensuring they receive the full benefits of physical activity.

Training my oldest client, Edith, remains one of the most memorable experiences in my career. Edith was living with Alzheimer's and relied on a wheelchair for mobility. Despite these challenges, the joy that our training sessions brought her was unmistakable. Each time I entered her room, I was greeted by her radiant smile—a clear indication of the positive impact our sessions had on her well-being. These moments underscored the profound connection that physical activity can foster, transcending mere exercise to touch the heart deeply. My journey with Edith took on an even more personal dimension when, pregnant with my first daughter, I had to temporarily pause our sessions. The hiatus lasted a few months following my daughter's birth. Upon resuming, I decided to bring my baby girl along for the visits. The introduction of my little angel to our sessions brought Edith an unparalleled level of happiness. It was as though the presence of a young child invigorated her spirit, bringing forth a wave of joy and vitality that was truly heartwarming to witness. These sessions with Edith evolved beyond physical training; they transformed into moments of genuine human connection and shared joy. Witnessing the positive effects of our sessions on Edith's mood and spirit was a powerful reminder of the holistic benefits of physical activity. It reinforced my belief in the importance of adaptability and personal connection in training, especially when working with seniors facing significant health challenges. Our time together was not only about maintaining physical health but also about enriching her quality of life, proving that the impact of thoughtful, compassionate training extends far beyond physical outcomes.

This profound experience illuminated a pivotal strategy I often employ with my clients: modifying exercises to accommodate their unique health needs, mainly by reducing the range of motion. For instance, for those who find deep bending challenging due to joint pain or osteoporosis, I recommend smaller, controlled movements that still stimulate the muscles without exerting undue stress on the bones. Providing stability with support aids like chairs or walls can also be incredibly beneficial. Additionally, pacing becomes essential for clients managing cardiovascular conditions. I make it a point to integrate rest periods within each session, allowing a moment for their heart rate to return to a steady state before progressing to the following exercise sequence.

Adapting exercises to meet individual needs and limitations is a cornerstone of creating an effective and safe workout regimen, especially for seniors. Here are detailed examples of how traditional exercises can be modified to accommodate various levels of mobility and health conditions, ensuring everyone can participate in and benefit from physical activity.

Seated Marches for Improved Leg Strength and Cardiovascular Health

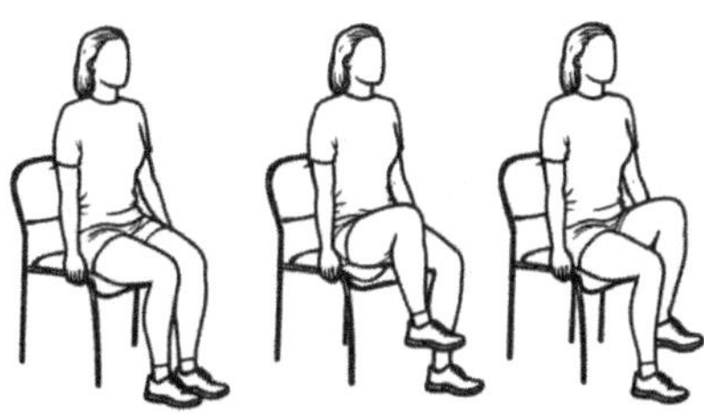

Seated marches present a secure alternative for those who find standing marches challenging due to balance concerns.

Begin this exercise by selecting a sturdy, armless chair and sitting at the edge with both feet planted firmly on the floor. This starting position ensures that your core is activated right from the outset, laying a solid foundation for the exercise. With your back straight and core engaged, lift one leg off the ground, bending at the knee to mimic the motion of marching. It's crucial to keep the movement controlled and deliberate to maximize muscle engagement. Alternate legs, maintaining a rhythmic pace that feels comfortable yet challenging. The goal is to lift your knees as high as your flexibility and comfort allow without straining. This seated variation does more than just build leg strength; it also stimulates your cardiovascular system, promoting heart health with minimal impact on your joints. By maintaining an upright posture throughout the exercise, you further enhance core stability and improve overall posture. The beauty of seated marches lies in their simplicity and effectiveness, making them a valuable addition to your balance and coordination workout regimen.

. **Wall Push-ups to Strengthen Upper Body with Reduced Joint Strain**

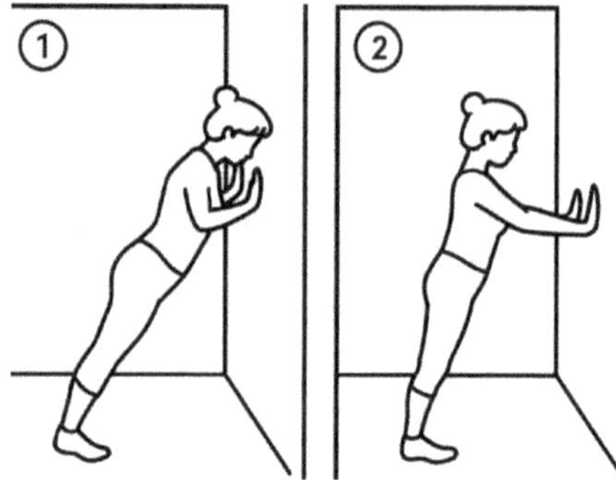

For individuals experiencing discomfort or limitations in their wrists or shoulders, engaging in traditional push-ups may pose a significant challenge, potentially exacerbating existing conditions. A practical and safe alternative to consider is the incorporation of wall push-ups into your exercise regimen. This modification allows for the engagement and strengthening of the chest, shoulders, and arms while significantly reducing undue stress on sensitive joints. To correctly execute a wall push-up, initiate the movement by positioning yourself approximately an arm's length away from a stable wall, ensuring your feet are planted shoulder-width apart for optimal stability. Carefully place your hands against the wall, aligning them with your shoulders to create a sturdy foundation for the movement. With your body in a straight line from head to heels, engage your core muscles to provide additional support throughout the exercise. Commence the push-up by slowly bending your elbows, allowing your body to approach the wall in a controlled manner. Pay close attention to maintaining a neutral spine, and avoid locking your elbows as you gently lower yourself. Once your face is near the wall, use the strength of your upper body to push back, returning to your starting position with your arms extended. The controlled movement not only targets the upper body muscles effectively but also ensures that the wrists and shoulders are spared from the high impact and strain associated with traditional, floor-based push-ups. Incorporating wall push-ups into your workout routine offers a practical solution for maintaining upper body strength without risking further injury to sensitive joints. This exercise is particularly beneficial for those seeking to enhance their fitness levels while managing conditions that limit their ability to perform high-impact exercises. By adjusting the distance of your feet from the wall, you can vary the difficulty of the exercise, making it suitable for a broad range of fitness levels and accommodating the progression of strength over time.

Chair Squats for Lower Body Strength Without the Risk of Falling

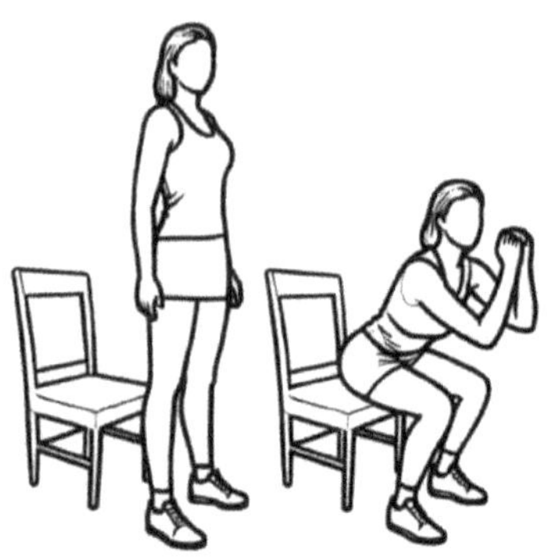

Chair squats offer an excellent modification for individuals who might find traditional standing squats challenging or who are concerned about balance and stability. To perform this exercise effectively, begin by positioning yourself in front of a sturdy chair, ensuring it is stable and won't slide away from you. Your feet should be set hip-width apart and firmly planted on the floor. Initiate the movement by engaging your core, keeping your chest lifted and your spine in a neutral position. This posture alignment is crucial as it ensures that the exercise targets the intended muscle groups while minimizing strain on your lower back. Slowly start to bend your knees, pushing your hips back as if you are about to sit down on the chair. It's essential to shift your weight into your heels, which helps activate the posterior chain muscles, including the glutes and hamstrings. Lower your body with control until you are just above the chair, hovering momentarily without actually making contact with the seat. This momentary pause increases muscle engagement, enhancing the strength-building aspect of the exercise. To return to the starting position, drive through your heels, pressing down into the floor to stand back up. This upward phase of the exercise further engages the thigh and buttock muscles, completing the movement. The presence of the chair serves not only as a guide for depth but also as a psychological safety net, significantly reducing the fear of falling backward.

This reassurance can encourage a deeper engagement in the exercise, as the risk of injury feels mitigated. For additional support, the exercise can be modified further by actually sitting down lightly on the chair before standing back up, which can be particularly beneficial for those just beginning to incorporate strength exercises into their routine or for individuals with severe balance issues. Incorporating chair squats into your workout regimen strengthens the thighs, hips, and buttocks while simultaneously improving balance and stability, making it a valuable exercise for enhancing overall functional fitness and independence.

****Toe Taps to Enhance Coordination and Lower Leg Strength****

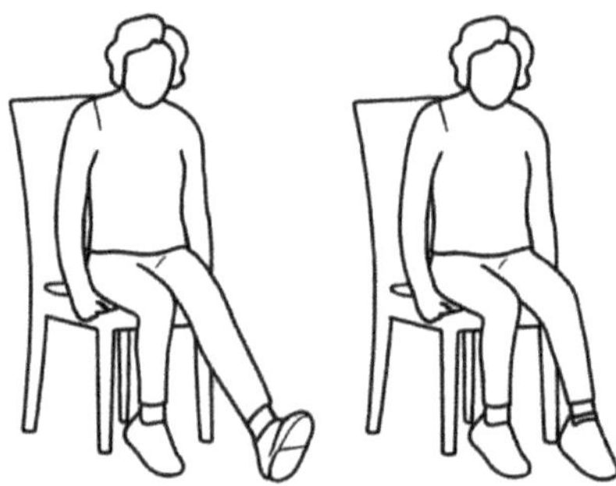

Sit comfortably in a sturdy, armless chair, ensuring your feet are flat on the floor and your spine is in a neutral position, promoting good posture. Gently extend your legs forward, allowing your heels to find a stable resting spot on the ground. Initiate the exercise by rhythmically tapping your toes against the floor, alternating between your left and right foot. This deliberate action not only activates the muscles in your lower legs but also encourages coordination between them. By focusing on the repetition and rhythm of the taps, you not only strengthen these essential muscles but also improve the neuromuscular connection, which is vital for maintaining walking stability and preventing falls. This exercise, with its simplicity and efficacy, is especially advantageous for individuals aiming to bolster their balance and enhance their overall mobility.

These tailored modifications exemplify the adaptability of exercises to accommodate the diverse physical needs and conditions of seniors, ensuring a pathway to fitness that prioritizes safety and efficacy. By weaving these adaptations into your daily routine, you can unlock a wealth of health benefits. Physical activity, tailored to their capabilities, fosters improved muscle strength and enhanced flexibility, laying the groundwork for heightened balance and coordination. This holistic approach significantly diminishes the likelihood of injuries, empowering seniors to lead active, fulfilling lives. Through careful adjustment and personalization of exercise routines, we can create a fitness landscape where every senior has the opportunity to thrive physically, demonstrating that with the proper modifications, the realm of physical wellness is accessible to all, regardless of age or mobility level.

As previously mentioned, it is wise to consult with health professionals if you do not have a personal trainer that is specialized in senior fitness, before starting a new exercise routine. They can provide insights tailored to your specific health conditions, ensuring your exercise plan is safe and effective.

Cool-Down and Recovery Tips

Transitioning your body from a heightened state of activity to a state of rest is very important for any exercise routine. This phase is essential for facilitating a smooth and gentle reduction in heart rate, allowing it to steadily return to its baseline level. This gradual process is crucial in averting the potential for dizziness or lightheadedness that can occur if the heart rate drops abruptly. Moreover, a well-structured cool-down phase aids in alleviating muscle stiffness by methodically relaxing the muscles, promoting flexibility, and minimizing the risk of discomfort or soreness in the aftermath of your workout.

To cool down effectively, you want to decrease your heart rate gradually to support circulation. A gentle-paced walk in place can accomplish this. Include some static stretching, focusing on your major muscle groups. Stretch your calves, quadriceps, hamstrings, shoulders, chest, and back, holding each stretch for 15 to 30 seconds. These stretches encourage muscle relaxation and enhance flexibility, helping your body shift seamlessly from active to resting.

** Standing calf stretch (Wall version)**

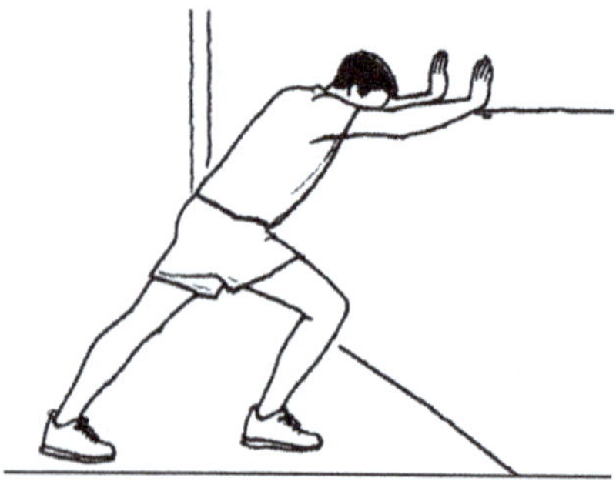

To perform a standing calf stretch at the wall, stand about arm's length from a sturdy wall and place your hands on it at chest height for support. Step one foot back about 1–2 feet, keeping it straight and flat on the floor, while the front foot remains closer to the wall with a slight bend in the knee. Lean your body gently toward the wall until you feel a stretch in the calf muscle of the back leg, ensuring the back heel stays pressed into the floor. Hold the stretch for 15–30 seconds, breathing deeply, then switch legs and repeat. Move slowly, avoid bouncing, and stop if you feel pain.

** Supported standing quad stretch **

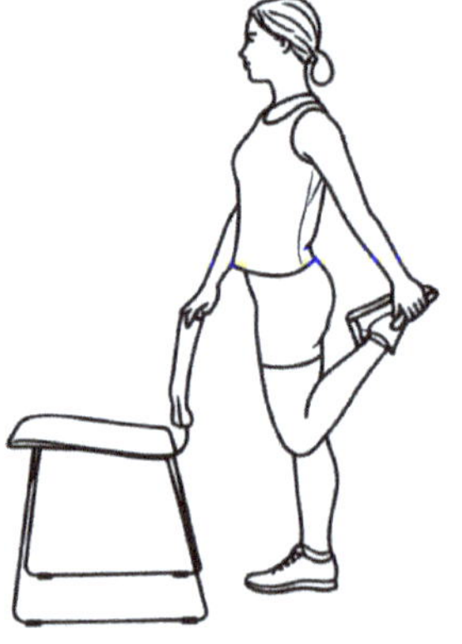

To perform a standing quad stretch using a chair for support, stand next to a sturdy chair and place one hand on it for balance. Bend one knee and lift your foot behind you, grabbing your ankle or the back of your foot with your free hand. Gently pull your foot toward your buttocks until you feel a stretch in the front of your thigh, keeping your knees close together and your back straight. Hold the stretch for 15–30 seconds, breathing deeply, then release and switch to the other leg. Move slowly, avoid pulling too hard, and use the chair for stability throughout.

** Seated hamstring stretch **

To perform a seated hamstring stretch, sit
on the edge of a sturdy chair with one foot
flat on the floor and the other leg extended
straight out in front of you, with your heel
resting on the floor and toes pointing up.
Keeping your back straight, gently lean forward from your hips toward the extended leg
until you feel a stretch in the back of your
thigh. Hold the stretch for 15–30 seconds,
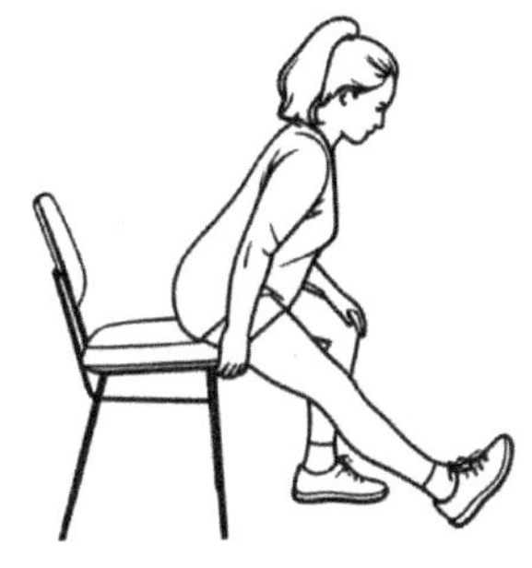
breathing deeply, then sit back up and switch to the other leg. Avoid rounding your back
and move slowly to prevent strain.

** Wall assisted chest stretch **

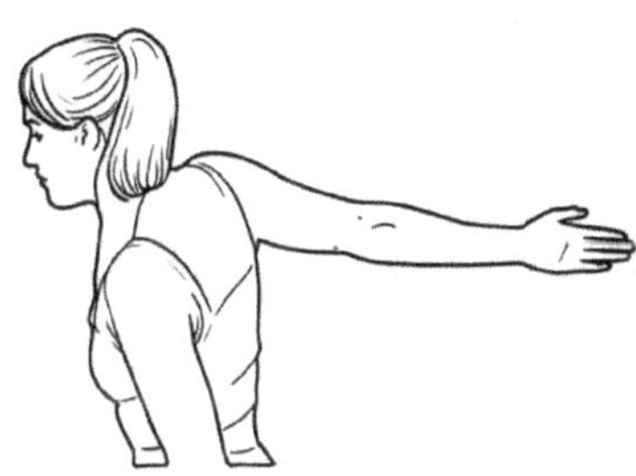
To perform a wall-assisted chest stretch, stand
next to a sturdy wall with your side facing it. Place
one hand on the wall at shoulder height, keeping
your arm straight. Slowly turn your body away
from the wall until you feel a gentle stretch across
your chest and the front of your shoulder. Hold
the stretch for 15–30 seconds, breathing deeply,
then relax and switch to the other side. Keep your movements slow and controlled, and
avoid overstretching to prevent strain.

** Tricep stretch **

To perform a tricep stretch, raise one arm overhead and bend your elbow so your hand reaches toward the middle of your upper back. Use your opposite hand to gently push your elbow back and down until you feel a stretch along the back of your upper arm. Hold the stretch for 15–30 seconds, breathing deeply, then switch to the other arm. Keep your back straight and avoid forcing the stretch to stay comfortable.

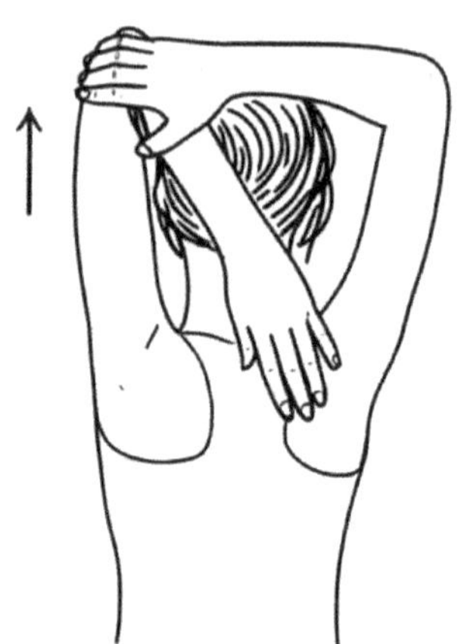

** Shoulder stretch **

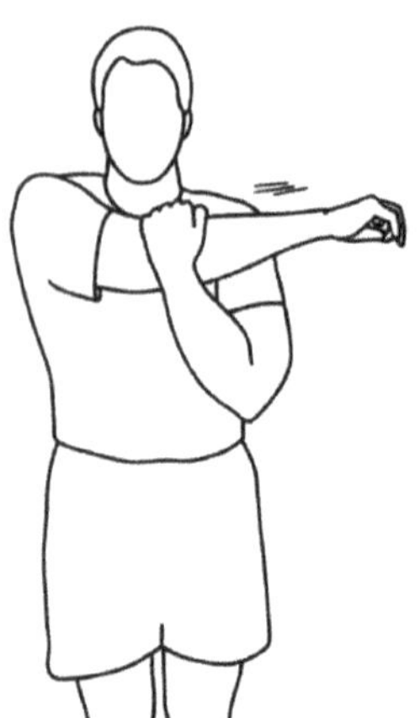

To perform a cross-body shoulder stretch, stand or sit tall with your back straight. Extend one arm straight across your chest at shoulder height. Use your opposite hand to gently pull the extended arm closer to your chest, keeping your shoulder relaxed. You should feel a stretch in the back of your shoulder. Hold the stretch for 15–30 seconds, breathing deeply, then switch to the other arm. Avoid twisting your torso or applying too much pressure.

Recovery

Recovery extends beyond the initial cool-down phase, reaching into the essential hours and days after your workout. This period is crucial for the body's recuperation process, emphasizing the importance of ongoing care following physical activity. Adequate hydration plays an indispensable role in this phase. Drinking water replenishes the fluids lost through perspiration and sustains all bodily functions, crucially including the process of muscle repair. The significance of proper nutrition in the recovery process cannot be overstated. Consuming a well-balanced meal that contains an optimal mix of proteins and carbohydrates is essential after exercising. This nutritional support provides your muscles with the necessary building blocks to repair, recover, and strengthen.

Incorporating sufficient rest into your exercise regimen is equally vital. Sleep serves as a foundational pillar of muscle recovery and overall health. During sleep, your body undergoes extensive repair and recovery processes. It's during these restful periods that muscles heal and adapt, bolstering their strength and resilience. Hence, integrating rest days into your workout schedule is critical, especially after engaging in intensive physical activities. This approach allows your muscles to recuperate and adjust, enhancing your physical capabilities over time.

Armed with these comprehensive strategies for safe exercise and recovery, we will now delve into specific exercises designed to bolster balance and coordination. These tailored exercises are foundational, empowering you to enhance your physical strength and independence, thereby enriching your quality of life.

3

PROGRESSIVE BALANCE EXERCISES

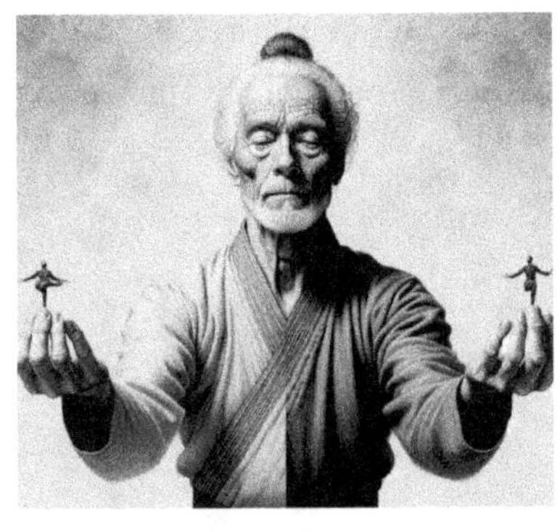

For those new to balance exercises, seated movements are a gateway to safely building foundational strength, setting the stage for more advanced activities later on. Seated balance exercises serve as a gentle introduction to the world of fitness. They offer the perfect blend of safety and challenge, allowing you to focus on building strength without fear of overexertion or injury. Practicing in a seated position significantly decreases the risk of falls, a concern that often accompanies starting a new exercise routine. These exercises help you develop foundational strength in a secure environment, laying the groundwork for more complex movements as you progress. They are not only about safety; they are about empowerment—giving you the tools to improve your balance at your own pace and on your own terms.

Below, we will explore a list of exercises specifically designed to fortify your strength, balance, and coordination from a seated position. These exercises are the stepping stones to a sturdier, more confident you. As you gradually master these movements and feel ready for more intensity, I invite you to delve into the advanced exercises presented in Chapter 8. This progression is designed with your growth in mind, ensuring a smooth transition as your capabilities expand.

However, it's crucial to listen to your body throughout this journey. If at any point you experience discomfort or find certain movements challenging, do not be disheartened.

Chapter 5 is dedicated to offering valuable modifications and alternatives to accommodate any limitations you may encounter. These adaptations ensure that you can continue to progress safely and comfortably, keeping your well-being paramount.

Maintaining proper posture and alignment during these exercises is vital for maximizing their benefits. Sit with your back straight, and remember to relax your shoulders. Avoid slumping or hunching. Imagine a string gently pulling you upwards from the crown of your head, encouraging a tall and proud posture. This posture will ensure that you perform the correct exercise while avoiding injury and also help you focus on the movement. By practicing good posture, you ensure that your exercises are effective and that you build strength in the right areas. It's a minor adjustment with a significant impact, reinforcing both your physical and mental well-being through mindful movement.

**Seated Ankle Circles to Enhance Lower Limb Flexibility **

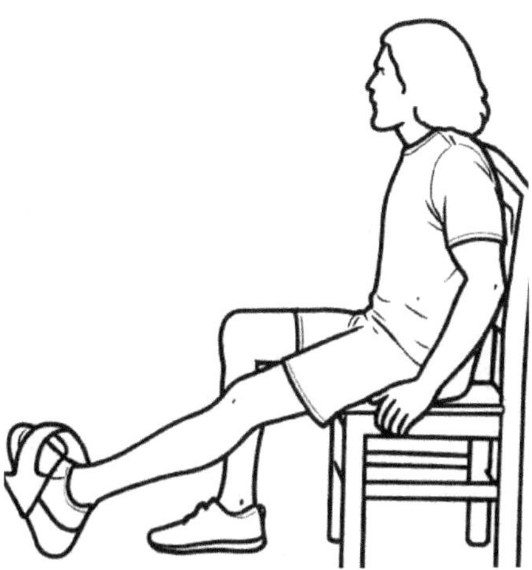

- While seated, extend one leg and rotate your ankle in a circular motion. You can rotate clockwise and then counterclockwise.

- This simple action improves flexibility in the lower limbs, enhancing your ability to move with ease and confidence.

- Both exercises can be performed daily, gradually increasing intensity as your strength builds.

Seated Marches for Improved Leg Strength and Cardiovascular Health

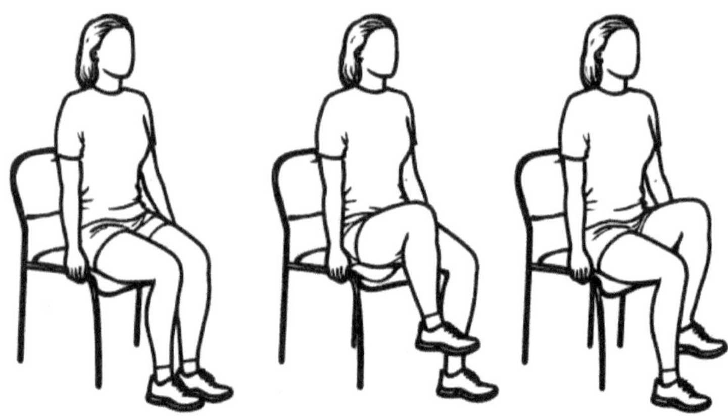

- While seated, lift one knee toward your chest in a marching motion, then lower it back down. Alternate legs to create a smooth rhythm.

- This simple yet effective exercise strengthens the lower body and improves co-ordination, enhancing your ability to move with ease and confidence.

- Both legs can be exercised alternately, and the activity can be performed daily. Start with small, controlled movements and gradually increase the height of your knee lifts or the speed of the march as your strength builds.

**** Seated Leg extension to Strengthen the Quads and improve Knee Stability & Balance ****

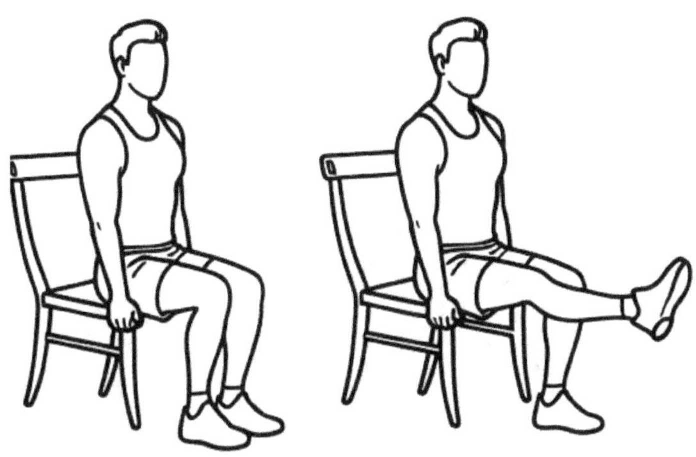

- While seated, extend one leg straight out in front of you until it is parallel to the floor or as high as is comfortable. Hold the position briefly, then lower your foot back down to the ground.

- Alternate legs to ensure both sides are worked equally. This simple action strengthens the quadriceps, improves knee stability, and enhances overall balance, contributing to a stronger and more confident lower body.

- This exercise can be performed daily, starting with slow, controlled movements. Gradually increase the duration of the hold or the number of repetitions as your strength and stability improve.

** Seated Shoulder Circles to Improve upper body Strength, Mobility & Coordination **

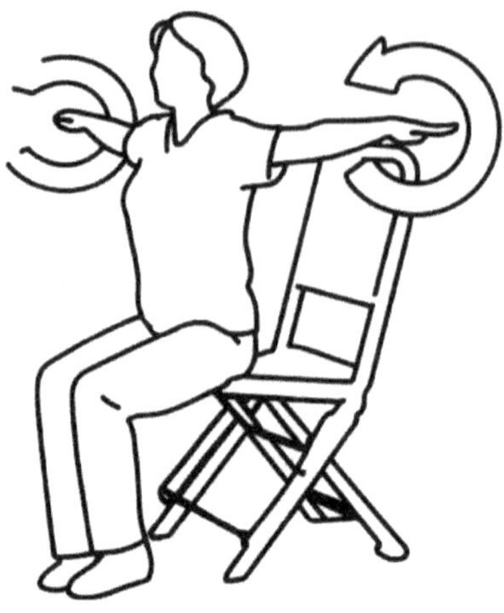

- Begin by rolling your shoulders in a circular motion. Move them forward, up, back, and down in a smooth, continuous motion. After several repetitions, reverse the direction, rolling your shoulders backward, up, forward, and down.

- This simple yet effective movement improves upper body strength, enhances shoulder mobility, and boosts coordination.

- This exercise can be performed daily, starting with small, gentle circles and gradually increasing the size of the motion as your flexibility and strength improve.

** Seated Shoulder Press to Build Upper Body Strength and Enhance Stability **

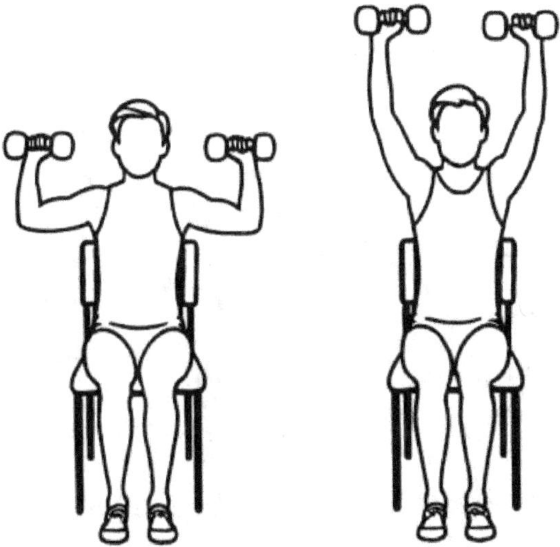

- While seated, start with your elbows bent and hands positioned at shoulder height, palms facing forward. Slowly press your arms upward until they are fully extended above your head. Pause briefly, then lower your arms back to the starting position.

- This movement strengthens the shoulders, improves upper body stability, and promotes better posture.

- This exercise can be performed daily, starting with light resistance or no weights. Gradually increase the resistance or the number of repetitions as your strength builds.

** Seated Chair Push-Up to Strengthen Arms, Shoulders, and Core **

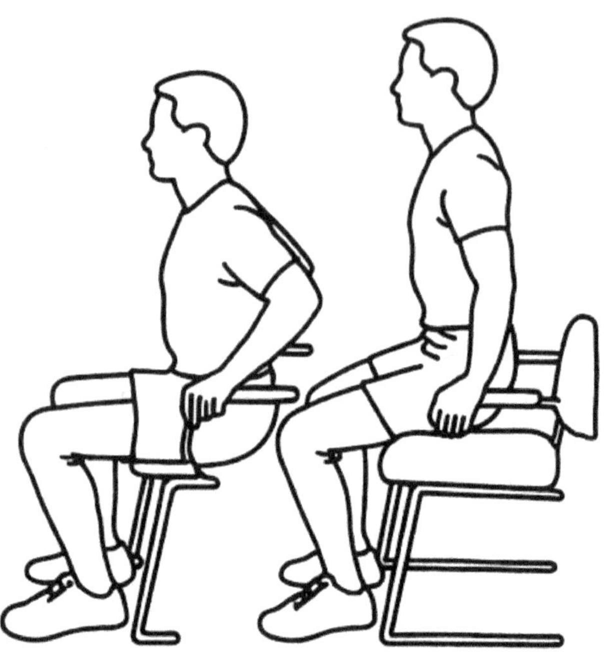

- While seated, place your hands on the armrests of your chair or the sides of the seat, ensuring your fingers are firmly gripping the edges. Engage your arms and shoulders to push your body upward, slightly lifting your hips off the seat. Hold briefly, then slowly lower yourself back down.

- This exercise strengthens your arms, shoulders, and core while also improving functional upper body strength.

- Perform this exercise daily, starting with small, controlled lifts. Gradually increase the height of the lift or the number of repetitions as your strength and endurance improve.

** Seated Calf Raise to Strengthen Calves and Improve Ankle Mobility **

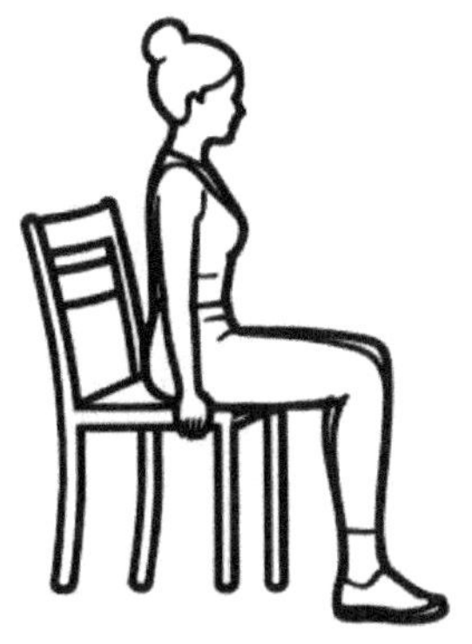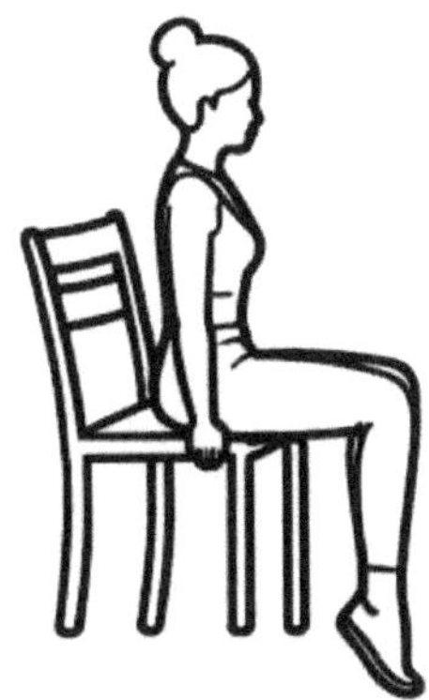

- While seated, keep your feet flat on the ground and knees at a 90-degree angle. Slowly lift your heels off the floor as high as possible, rising onto the balls of your feet. Hold briefly, then lower your heels back to the ground.

- This movement strengthens your calf muscles and enhances ankle mobility, supporting better balance and lower body stability.

- This exercise can be performed daily. Start with slow, controlled movements, and gradually increase the number of repetitions or add light resistance, such as placing your hands on your thighs, as your strength improves.

4

⸺ ❖ ⸺

HOLISTIC HEALTH AND MINDFULNESS

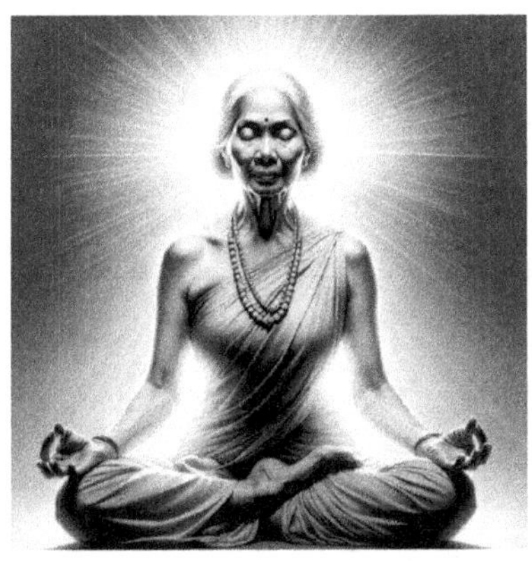

My years of teaching Yoga have helped me truly connect with myself, and I often incorporate it into my training programs. It has taught me how to find a balance between my mind and body. The essence of mindfulness is a practice that invites you to be fully present in each moment, particularly in the context of fitness, which can enhance your physical performance and overall health. By focusing your attention on the present and cultivating a more profound awareness of your body and its movements, you can perform exercises with precision and intention, reducing the likelihood of injury and increasing the efficiency of your workout.

For seniors, the benefits of mindfulness in fitness are particularly significant. It offers an avenue for improving concentration and mental clarity. Training your mind to focus boosts your cognitive functions, enhancing your ability to engage fully in activities. Mindfulness also fosters emotional resilience, providing a buffer against stress as it encourages a mindset of acceptance and patience.

Integrating mindfulness into daily life doesn't require complex techniques or significant time commitments. Simple practices like mindful breathing exercises can be a powerful starting point. Take a moment each day to sit quietly. Focus on the natural rhythm of your breath. Inhale deeply through your nose, place one hand on your belly, and feel it expand, then exhale slowly through your mouth. This practice anchors you in the present, calming your mind and body. Similarly, a body scan meditation can enhance your awareness of physical sensations. Lie comfortably and mentally scan your body from head to toe, noting any areas of tension or ease.

Mindfulness Exercise: Body Scan Practice

Begin by finding a serene spot where you have the option to either sit in a comfortable chair or lie down on a soft surface. Ensure this area is free from distractions to fully immerse yourself in the exercise. Once settled, gently close your eyes and allow yourself to take several deep breaths—inhale slowly through your nose, letting your chest and belly rise, and then exhale gradually through your mouth, feeling a sense of release with each breath.

As you continue to breathe deeply, shift your focus to your feet. Notice any sensations you might feel. It could be a slight tingling, a sense of warmth, or even the weight of your feet against the ground or your socks. Acknowledge these sensations without any judgment, simply observing them as they are.

Gradually, let your awareness ascend through your body. Move from your feet to your calves, pausing to feel any sensations there. Continue this process slowly, traveling up to your knees, thighs, and hips. Take your time to really tune into each part of your body, recognizing how each area might feel different.

When you reach your abdomen, pay attention to the rise and fall with each breath. Notice the gentle expansion and contraction, and the sensation of breathing that connects you to the moment. Continue moving your awareness upwards—through your chest, shoulders, and neck. If at any point your mind begins to wander, acknowledge this gently without criticism, and guide your focus back to the part of the body you were concentrating on.

This mindful body scan not only promotes relaxation but also deepens your connection with your body. It enhances your awareness and mindfulness, crucial components for improving balance and coordination. By regularly practicing this exercise, you'll cultivate a greater understanding of your body's signals and how to respond to them, ultimately contributing to your overall stability and wellbeing.

Breathing Techniques for Relaxation

Breathing is a powerful tool, often overlooked in its simplicity and effectiveness. How we breathe can significantly impact our nervous system, influencing our stress levels and overall sense of calm. By focusing on controlled breathing, you can activate the parasympathetic nervous system. This system is responsible for the "rest and digest" state. This system helps lower your heart rate and blood pressure, creating a sense of tranquility that permeates throughout your body. Imagine the soothing sensation of a gentle wave washing over you, lulling your nerves into a state of peace. This calming effect reduces tension and allows your mind and body to relax, providing a foundation for greater well-being and resilience.

Learning specific breathing techniques can be a gateway to profound relaxation and focus. One such technique is diaphragmatic breathing, often referred to as belly breathing. For this, you will need to find a comfortable position, sitting or lying down, and place one hand on your chest and the other on your belly. Take a slow, deep breath through your nose, allowing your belly to expand as it fills with air. Exhale slowly and feel your belly deflate. This exercise encourages deep relaxation by fully engaging the diaphragm, which increases the amount of oxygen entering your lungs.

Another technique is box breathing, which promotes focus and reduces stress. Picture a box as you breathe. This rhythmic pattern helps steady the mind and body, creating a sense of balance and calm.

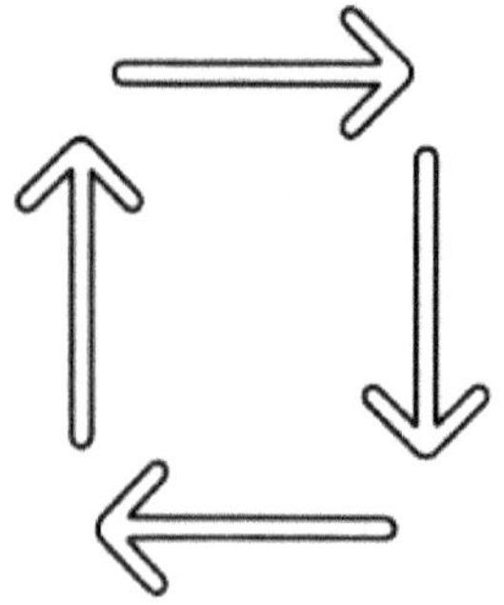

1- Inhale for a count of four.

2- Hold your breath for four.

3- Exhale for four.

4- Pause for four before repeating.

The physiological benefits of effective breathing extend beyond relaxation. Effective breathing can contribute to improved physical health. By enhancing oxygen delivery to your muscles, controlled breathing supports optimal muscle function and endurance. This means your muscles receive the energy they need to perform efficiently, reducing fatigue and enhancing performance. Additionally, regular practice of breathing exercises can improve lung capacity and efficiency. This increased capacity allows you to take in more oxygen with each breath, supporting cardiovascular health and increasing your stamina. Over time, these benefits can lead to improved overall fitness and resilience, making breathing exercises a valuable component of your health routine.

Incorporating breathing exercises into your daily life is both simple and rewarding. Try starting your day with a morning breathing ritual. Take five minutes each morning to engage in diaphragmatic breathing, setting a calm and focused tone for the day ahead. These moments of stillness can be a powerful way to ground yourself.

Mindful Movement and Awareness

Imagine walking through a peaceful park, each step deliberate and meaningful. This is mindful movement, where the focus is on the quality of each motion. It's about being aware of how the body moves, ensuring that every action is purposeful. In fitness, this approach enhances the connection between the mind and body, transforming routine exercises into experiences that engage both physical and mental faculties. When you pay attention to how your foot lands or how your arm swings, you not only improve your technique but also deepen your relationship with your own body. This awareness can elevate an ordinary walk into a practice of mindfulness, where every step is an opportunity to explore and appreciate your body's capabilities.

Mindful movement plays a crucial role in injury prevention. By being aware of your body's alignment, you reduce the risk of strains or pulls. Instead of pushing through discomfort, you must learn to listen to your body's signals, making necessary changes that protect your joints and muscles.

Viewing exercise as a holistic practice brings a host of benefits. When you integrate breathing with movement, you create a flow that supports both physical and mental well-being. Breathing deeply and rhythmically during exercise boosts oxygen delivery to your muscles, enhancing performance and endurance. During exercises, I frequently remind my clients about the importance of maintaining steady breathing. It's natural to hold our breath during challenging moments, but mastering deliberate breathing is crucial for overcoming these hurdles. The power of breathwork cannot be overstated, as it is a critical factor in achieving our fitness goals.

Nutrition Tips for Optimal Health

Nutrition is not just about satisfying hunger; it's the cornerstone of health, especially as we age. I experienced firsthand the profound impact an unhealthy diet can have on one's lifestyle. Following the conclusion of my gymnastics career, I found myself grappling with a weight gain of 50 pounds. This marked a significant shift from the strict fitness and nutritional routines I followed as an athlete, where maintaining a lean physique was not just encouraged but required. This transition exposed a gap in my understanding; I had yet to anticipate the challenge of reverting to a healthy lifestyle after years of structured training and dieting. The realization hit hard—it's a daunting task to regain control of one's health, but it's far from impossible. The turning point came when I was diagnosed with rheumatoid arthritis. This diagnosis was a wake-up call, prompting me to overhaul my lifestyle, starting with my diet. Relearning how to nourish my body was a journey that involved understanding the balance of macronutrients, the importance of whole foods, and the role of hydration. This period of transformation was not just about weight loss; it was about reclaiming my health and vitality, one meal at a time. Through this journey, I successfully shed 65 pounds by embracing a healthier lifestyle and deepening my understanding of nutrition and fitness.

A balanced diet fuels your body, supporting energy levels and aiding recovery after physical activities. Think of macronutrients—carbohydrates, proteins, and fats—as the building blocks your body needs to function optimally.

Carbohydrates provide the quick energy necessary for exercise, while proteins play a critical role in muscle repair and growth. Fats, often misunderstood, are essential for hormone production and cell health. Vitamins and minerals, though needed in smaller quantities, are equally vital. They ensure muscle health and overall vitality. For instance, magnesium helps with muscle function, while iron is crucial for transporting oxygen through the bloodstream.

For seniors, dietary recommendations often focus on maintaining bone health and reducing inflammation. Incorporating anti-inflammatory foods like berries, leafy greens, and fatty fish can help manage inflammation, which is expected as we age. These foods are rich in antioxidants and omega-3 fatty acids, which support your immune system and reduce joint pain. Calcium and vitamin D are essential for bone health. Dairy products, fortified plant milks, and leafy greens are excellent sources of calcium. Vitamin D, which helps your body absorb calcium, can be found in fortified foods and through safe sun exposure. Ensuring you get enough of these nutrients can help maintain bone density and reduce the risk of fractures, allowing you to remain active and independent.

Planning meals that support your fitness goals doesn't have to be complicated. Start by creating balanced plates with adequate protein, healthy fats, and a variety of fruits and vegetables. This approach ensures you get a great variety of nutrients. Consider timing your meals around your exercise routine. Eating a small meal or snack with carbohydrates and protein about an hour before exercising can provide the energy you need and support muscle recovery afterward. Think of a banana with nut butter or yogurt with berries as quick, nutritious options. These strategies help maximize your energy levels and improve your exercise performance, making each workout more effective.

You will find a sample meal plan in the following pages which provides a balanced approach, incorporating a variety of nutrients to support your health and fitness.

Sample Meal Plan

Breakfast: Oatmeal with diced apple and a sprinkle of cinnamon.

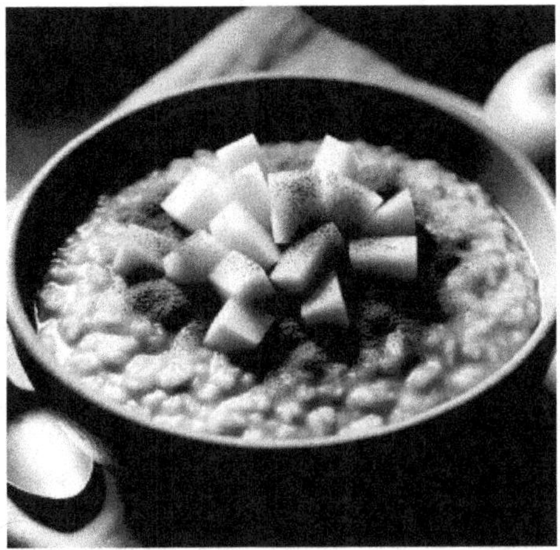

Snack: Greek yogurt with a handful of walnuts.

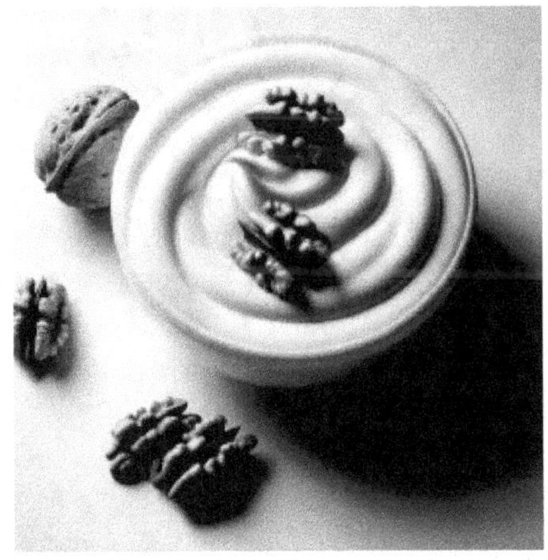

Lunch: Grilled chicken wrap with mixed greens, cherry tomatoes, and olive oil dressing.

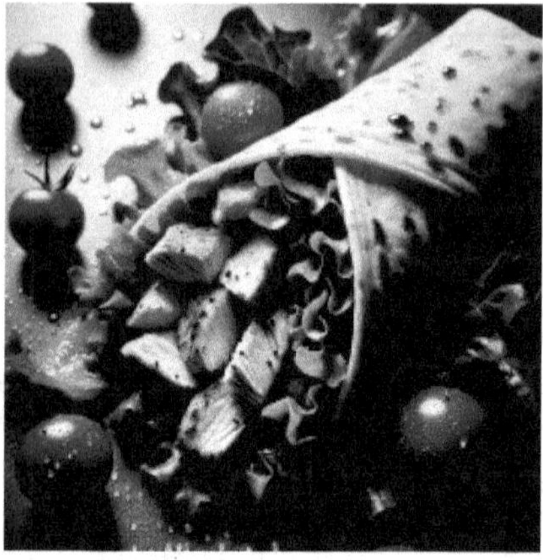

Snack: A small serving of hummus with carrot sticks.

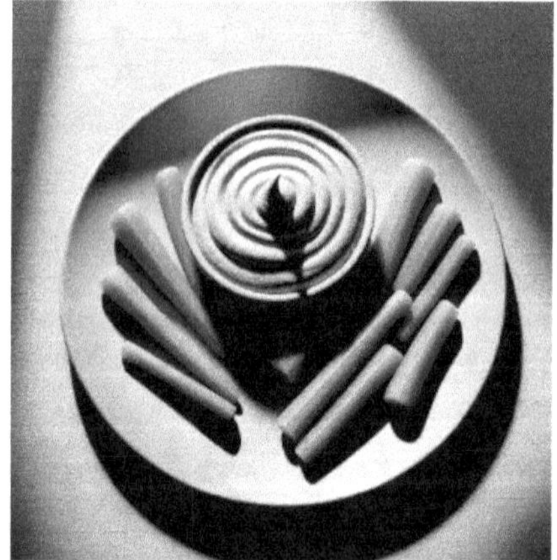

Dinner: Baked salmon with quinoa and steamed broccoli.

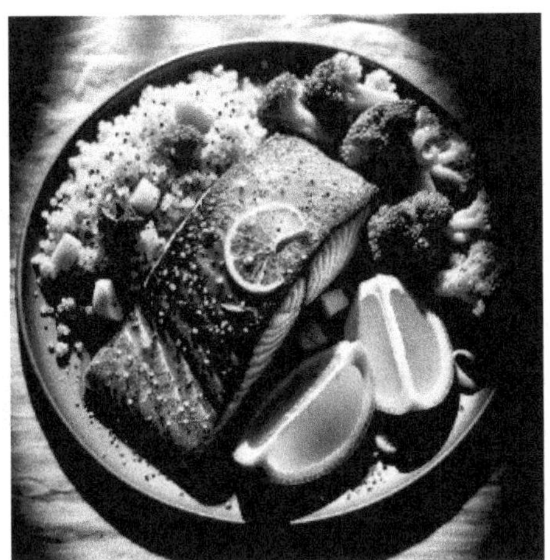

Hydration and Its Impact on Mobility

Proper hydration is more than just quenching thirst; it's a fundamental aspect of physical health, directly impacting mobility and joint function. When you're well-hydrated, your joints are lubricated, which allows for smoother and pain-free movement. This lubrication reduces friction between the bones, minimizing discomfort and the risk of injury during physical activities. Moreover, hydration helps regulate your body temperature, especially during exercise. As you engage in physical activities, your body generates heat, and sweating is your natural cooling mechanism. Adequate water intake ensures that you can sweat effectively, preventing overheating and fatigue.

Maintaining optimal hydration is pivotal, and following straightforward guidelines can be beneficial. It's recommended that seniors consume approximately eight cups (2,000 ml) of water daily. For those who may not favor plain water, opting for herbal teas or infusing water with natural flavors can be delightful alternatives, making it more appealing to meet daily hydration targets.

Maintaining hydration can become more challenging as we age. Certain medications can affect hydration levels, either by increasing fluid loss or altering thirst perception. Understanding these challenges is vital to developing effective hydration strategies. By being proactive, you can counteract these effects and ensure that your body remains well-hydrated, supporting both your physical and cognitive functions.

Implementing effective strategies is essential for maintaining consistent hydration. My personal journey with hydration has taught me the value of utilizing hydration reminder apps, a simple yet powerful tool to ensure I meet my daily water intake. Juggling the responsibilities of being both a full-time mother and a professional, I've found these reminders to be a practical solution for staying hydrated. This approach not only aids in meeting my hydration goals but also enhances my mobility and overall health, empowering me to take charge of my well-being amidst a busy lifestyle.

Creating a Balanced Wellness Routine

Establishing a balanced wellness regimen is crucial for embarking and maintaining this journey toward health. This process requires patience and a willingness to experiment as you identify the routines that work best with your personal lifestyle.

For myself, pre-planning my meals for the entire week has helped me achieve this balance. Training in the early morning, before my mom and work obligations kick in, is what I found to work best to maintain my fitness routine and feel energized throughout the day. The surge of energy I experience post-exercise is invaluable, especially when it comes time to play with my children. My energy levels have also sparked curiosity among other fellow moms. I frequently get asked, "Where do you get your energy?" My response is straightforward: "I work out!" This simple yet effective routine of morning exercise not only boosts my physical stamina but also contributes profoundly to my mental and emotional health.

Exercise invigorates the body, keeping muscles strong and joints flexible. Nutrition fuels your body, providing the necessary energy and nutrients to support an active lifestyle.

Mindfulness enriches your mental and emotional well-being, allowing you to navigate challenges with greater resilience and clarity. Combining these elements forms a thorough approach to health that addresses all aspects of your life.

It is essential to make this a priority; it is vital to take a moment to reflect on what you hope to achieve. Perhaps you want to maintain your independence, enhance your energy levels, or simply find more joy in daily activities. Defining these goals provides direction and purpose. Once you've established your objectives, the next step is to schedule it in. Set time aside each day for exercise, whether a brisk morning walk or a gentle evening stretch. Incorporate nutritious meals into your routine, planning ahead to ensure you have healthy options available. Mindfulness practices, such as meditation, can be woven into your day to support mental clarity and emotional balance. By creating a structured plan, you cultivate a routine that supports your overall well-being. Structure, I have found, is the key to success.

Understanding the fluctuating nature of our physical and mental needs is essential. Some days may bring a surge of energy, making it the perfect time for a vigorous workout. On less energetic days, a calm walk or some rest might serve you better. My experience has underscored the importance of tuning into my body's signals. Whether I'm feeling energetic or more subdued, I adapt my activity level accordingly, respecting my body's current state. This approach is a powerful affirmation of your dedication to wellness, promoting consistency in your health routine.

As you embark on your journey toward improved well-being, it is important to focus on practical ways to incorporate a balanced wellness routine, emphasizing the integration of exercise, nutrition, and mindfulness principles into your daily life. By assessing your personal health goals and scheduling regular activities, you cultivate a routine that supports long-term health and independence. This holistic approach enhances your quality of life, reducing the risk of chronic disease and empowering you to live each day with energy and joy. As we move forward, the next chapter will delve into the specifics of implementing these practices, offering practical tips and strategies to help you thrive.

5

ADDRESSING COMMON PHYSICAL LIMITATIONS

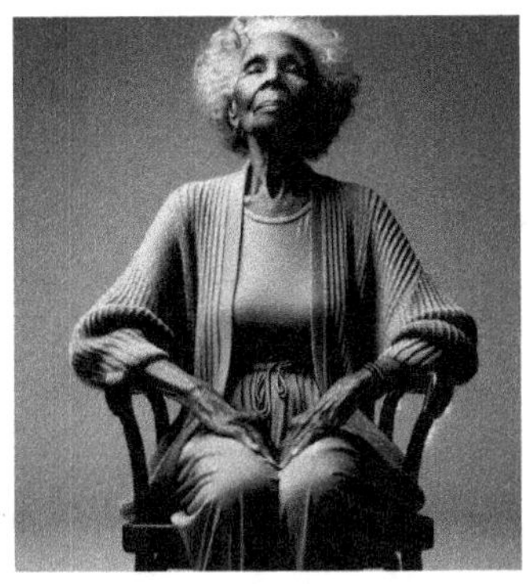

My grandmother frequently awakens to the discomfort of stiff joints. Arthritis can be a silent thief of joy, affecting mobility and independence. It creeps into the joints, often targeting the hands, knees, hips, and spine, bringing pain and stiffness that can make the simplest of tasks feel daunting. But this doesn't have to be the narrative of your day. Understanding arthritis and its impact on your body is the first step toward reclaiming your mobility and enhancing your quality of life.

Arthritis affects the joints by causing inflammation, which leads to pain and stiffness. This inflammation can limit your range of motion and make it difficult to perform everyday activities. The hands, knees, and hips are commonly affected, areas pivotal to movement and dexterity. Joint pain can vary from a mild ache to intense discomfort, which can fluctuate with changes in weather or activity levels. The stiffness, often worse in the morning or after periods of inactivity, can seem immobilizing. But there is hope, and that hope lies in movement. Exercise, especially low-impact routines, can be a powerful antidote to the limitations arthritis imposes.

On those days when a peaceful moment of relief is sought, engaging in simple, joint-friendly exercises can significantly impact your well-being. Take finger stretches, for example, which effectively enhance hand dexterity and alleviate stiffness. Begin by spreading your fingers as wide as possible before gently bringing each fingertip to your thumb, forming an "O" shape.

An especially memorable experience involved my client Edith, who suffered from severe arthritis, causing her hands to clench shut painfully. We saw remarkable improvement through consistently practicing these stretches; her hands gradually opened, restoring her ability to grasp objects. This progress was so impactful that her caretaker learned the routine, ensuring Edith could maintain her practice daily, even in my absence. Consistency is the cornerstone of managing arthritis effectively. Regular exercise helps keep the joints flexible, enhancing the muscles around them and strengthening them. This alone will help reduce pain and improve function. It's about making movement a part of your daily routine. By maintaining an active lifestyle, you take control of your health, empowering yourself to live with greater freedom and less discomfort. Remember, each movement is a step toward a stronger, more resilient you.

Improving Flexibility with Gentle Stretches

Flexibility is like the oil that keeps the engine of our bodies running smoothly. As we age, maintaining flexibility becomes even more important, offering a greater range of motion in everyday activities and reducing the risk of injury. I was blessed to have learned so many flexibility techniques as a gymnast, personal trainer, and yoga instructor. I am able to guide my clients in these techniques to keep them nimble and active.

When flexibility is nurtured, it allows for fluid movements, making your daily tasks easier. Increased flexibility is an asset to have in your pocket as it prevents falls, which is a major concern as we age, enabling us to recover our balance quickly if we stumble. It acts as a safeguard, ensuring that our bodies respond swiftly and efficiently to unexpected movements with less chance of injury. I strongly advocate incorporating gentle stretching routines into your daily life. These do not require a gym or special equipment, just time and attention.

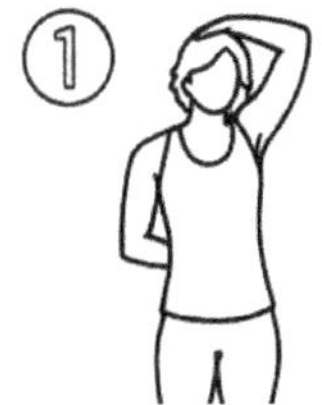
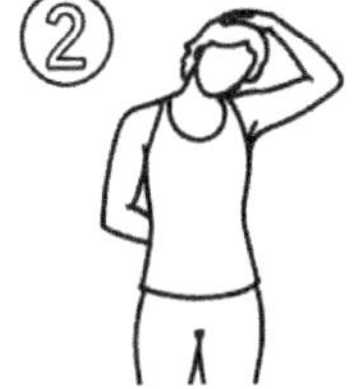

Neck stretches can provide significant relief from tension. Start by sitting comfortably, letting your shoulders drop, and slowly tilting your head to one side, feeling the stretch along the opposite side of your neck. Hold this position for a few breaths before switching sides.

The cat-cow stretch is another dynamic movement excellent for spine flexibility. Begin on your hands and knees, arching your back towards the ceiling like a cat and then drop your belly to the floor while lifting your head and tailbone towards the sky. This stretch enhances spinal mobility and sig-

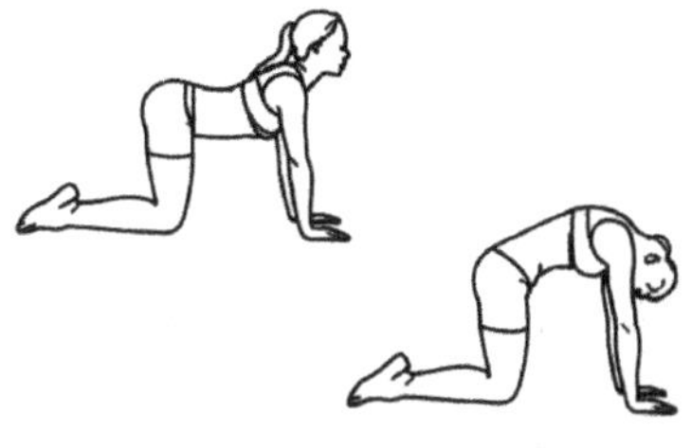

nificantly reduces back stiffness, facilitating smoother, more comfortable movements throughout the day. It's a vital part of my daily regimen, specifically tailored to manage my degenerative disk disease, keeping my spine flexible and functional. Interestingly, this exercise is adaptable for various mobility levels.

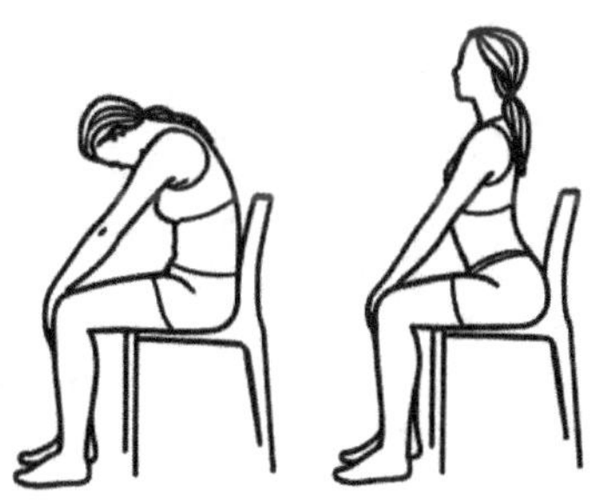

For instance, my 95-year-old grandmother modifies the cat-cow stretch to perform it seated on a chair, accommodating her physical needs while still benefiting from the exercise's Core and spinal engagement.

Remarkably, despite her age, she maintains enough mobility and strength to play on the floor with my children. Her ability to stay active and vibrant, engaging in playful interactions at 95, is a profound source of inspiration and a testament to the adaptability and effectiveness of these exercises across generations.

Another important aspect of stretching is the breath work. When stretching, focus on your breathing—inhale deeply before you begin the stretch, and exhale slowly as you move into the position. This helps relax your muscles and will also help achieve a deeper stretch. Hold each stretch for 15 to 30 seconds, maintaining a gentle tension without bouncing, as bouncing can lead to injuries. The stretch should feel comfortable and soothing, not painful. Repeat each stretch three times, gradually increasing the duration of the stretch as your flexibility improves. Try to aim to hold a stretch for one minute. However, it is crucial to listen to your body to avoid injuries. If a stretch feels too intense, ease back until it's comfortable.

Understanding Your Flexibility Needs

- Identify Areas of Tension: Reflect on parts of your body that feel stiff or tense. Where do you notice the most discomfort during daily activities?

- Set Flexibility Goals: Consider what you hope to achieve through stretching. Is it more effortless movement, pain relief, or simply a moment of relaxation?

- Create a Stretching Plan: Dedicate a specific time each day to stretch. Consistency is vital to seeing improvement.

- Note Your Progress: Keep a journal of your stretching routine, noting any changes in flexibility or comfort. Celebrate small victories in movement and mobility.

Flexibility is a journey that can be tailored to fit your individual needs and lifestyle. By embracing gentle stretches, you invite more freedom and ease into your movements, enhancing your overall well-being.

Strengthening the Core for Better Balance

When we think of the Core, we imagine the abdominal muscles. However, it is much more than this. It's the body's powerhouse. It is a complex group of muscles that includes the abdomen, lower back, hips, and pelvis muscles, which form a central support base, stabilizing the body and enabling movement with ease. A strong core plays one of the most significant roles in strength, balance and stability. It absorbs shocks and provides support, ensuring that your body remains steady and aligned. This stability is crucial in preventing falls, a concern as we age. In addition, Core strength enhances Posture. When your core muscles are robust, they support your spine and pelvis, allowing you to move with confidence, all while reducing the risk of injury. Simple exercises performed regularly can yield significant benefits. Seated torso twists are an excellent way to engage the obliques, the muscles on the sides of your waist that assist in rotation and stability.

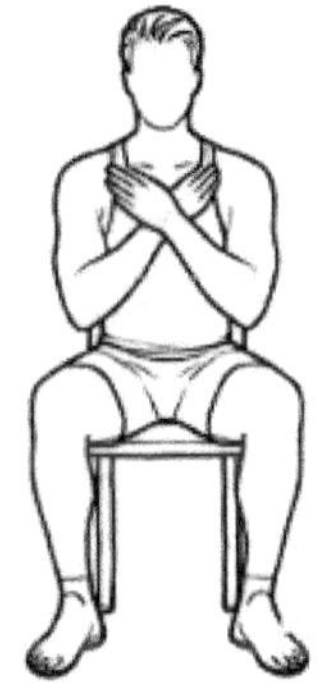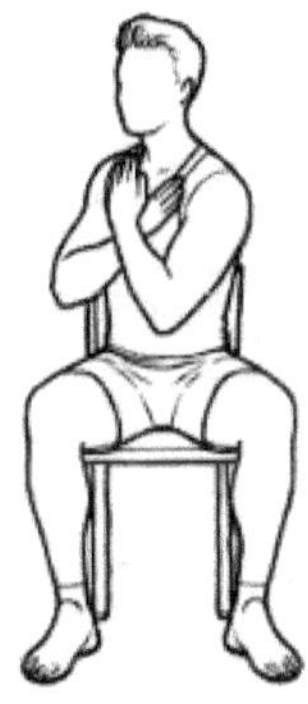

Sit upright in a chair with your feet flat on the floor. Cross your arms over your chest and gently twist your torso to one side, hold for a moment, then return to the center before twisting to the other side. This exercise not only strengthens the obliques but also improves flexibility in the spine, supporting daily movements like turning and reaching.

Another effective exercise is leg lifts, which target the lower abdominal muscles. While seated, extend your legs straight out in front of you, then lift them a few inches off the ground. Hold briefly before lowering them back down. You can modify this exercise by lifting one leg at a time for additional stability. This movement engages the lower abs, which is crucial for stability and balance.

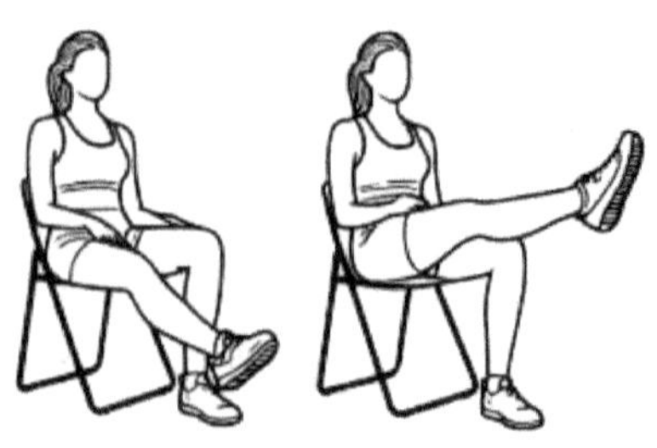

Everyone's fitness level is different, and it's essential to tailor exercises to suit your abilities. If you're new to core exercises or find them challenging, it would be helpful to use a chair. For those who struggle with flexibility or strength, reducing the range of motion in exercises is another effective modification. Instead of lifting legs high during leg lifts, try smaller, more controlled movements while holding them for each repetition. Time under tension does matter, and I use this approach with my clients at every session. This approach allows you to gradually build strength, minimizing the risk of injury while benefiting from the exercise.

Progression is key in any exercise routine, and core strengthening is no exception. Start with basic exercises and gradually increase the intensity as your strength improves. Set weekly goals to guide your progress, such as adding an extra set of repetitions or holding positions longer. This steady increase in intensity encourages muscle growth and endurance, leading to greater core stability over time. Monitoring your improvements can provide motivation and insight into your progress. Take note of how long you can hold each exercise or how many repetitions you can perform, and track these metrics regularly. Seeing your progress documented can be incredibly rewarding.

Strengthening your Core is about enhancing your overall quality of life. With a strong core, you can move through your day more easily and confidently, participating in activities you enjoy without fearing falls or injury. It supports your independence, allowing you to engage fully with the world around you. As you incorporate these exercises into your routine, remember that consistency is your greatest ally. Each small step contributes to a stronger, more stable you, empowering you to live life on your terms.

Tailoring Workouts for Limited Mobility

Facing the challenges of limited mobility can feel daunting, mainly when these challenges restrict your exercise options. Common issues include difficulty standing for extended periods, making traditional workouts seem overwhelming. The fatigue accompanying prolonged standing often leads to discouragement, creating a cycle where inactivity exacerbates the problem.

Limited joint motion is another hurdle, as stiffness can prevent you from fully participating in exercises that require a broad range of movement. These restrictions can sap your confidence, making the thought of starting any fitness regimen intimidating. However, it's important to remember that there are strategies and modifications available that enable you to stay active and maintain your health. You just have to start and trust in the process.

Seated exercise routines offer a practical solution for maintaining physical activity accessible, ensuring that individuals of any mobility level can participate.

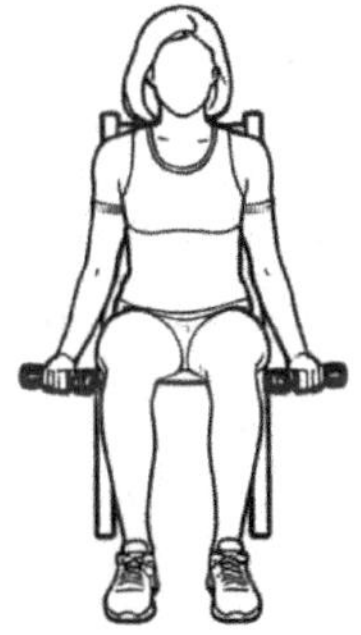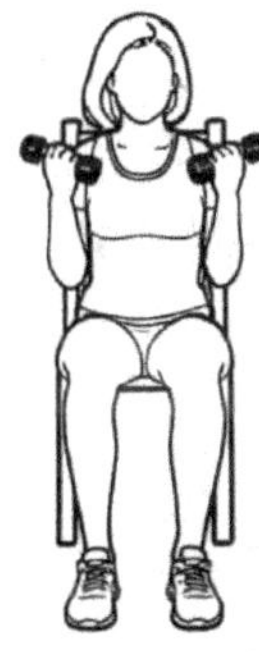

For example, seated arm curls are an excellent method for enhancing upper body strength without necessitating standing. Sitting in a chair with a straight back and lifting lightweight dumbbells or resistance bands, one can curl the weights toward the shoulders and then lower them gradually, engaging the biceps effectively.

This particular movement not only fortifies the arms but also improves the capacity for performing everyday tasks such as lifting and carrying. Additionally, exercises like shoulder circles and chair pushups can be executed while seated, allowing for a comprehensive upper-body regimen that targets both major and minor muscle groups, all from the comfort of a chair.

Personalization is vital when it comes to exercise, especially for those with limited mobility. Consult with healthcare providers to develop a personalized plan that addresses your specific needs and goals. If you choose to work with a personal trainer, it is best to ensure they have their certifications and experience in training clients with limited mobility. They can offer guidance on which exercises are suitable and how to perform them correctly. They can also assist in tracking your progress and making adjustments as needed.

Managing Back Pain During Exercise

Back pain frequently affects seniors, influencing daily activities and exercise habits. Personally, I navigate this challenge by adapting my routines based on the intensity of back pain experienced on any given day. Interestingly, I've observed a noticeable improvement in my condition on days filled with activity compared to those spent with less movement.

Degenerative conditions such as osteoporosis further complicate matters, causing bones to become brittle and fragile, increasing the risk of fractures. The spine, in particular, is susceptible to compression fractures, which can lead to persistent pain and a stooped posture. These changes not only affect your physical health but also your confidence and independence. The fear of pain or injury can deter you from engaging in activities you once enjoyed, leading to a more sedentary lifestyle that exacerbates the problem. Understanding these underlying causes of back pain is essential for managing symptoms and finding relief.

One of the more common pain points is back pain. In order to combat back pain and promote spine health, it's important to incorporate exercises that target the lower back and improve flexibility. If you are able to lie on the floor, bridges are a great starting point.

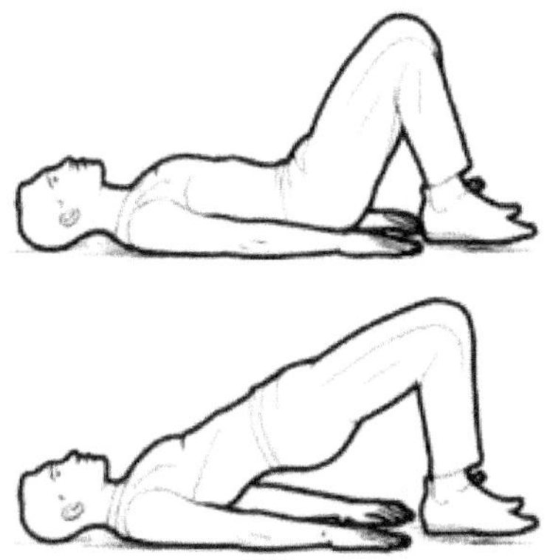

Lie on your back with your knees bent and feet flat on the floor. Slowly lift your hips towards the ceiling, squeezing your glutes and engaging your Core. Hold for a few seconds before gently lowering your hips back to the ground. This exercise strengthens the lower back and hamstring muscles, providing stability and support for your spine.

For those who find it challenging to lie on the floor, performing pelvic tilts while standing or seated can be highly advantageous. This exercise gently encourages you to press your lower back against a surface, aiming to align your spine vertically, thus minimizing the arch. This is accomplished 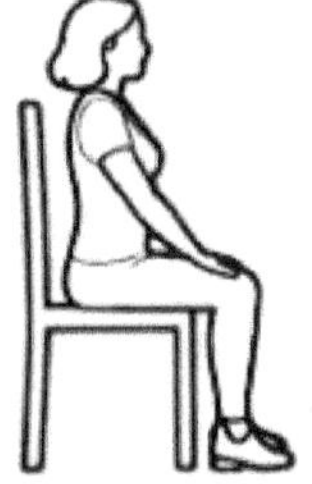 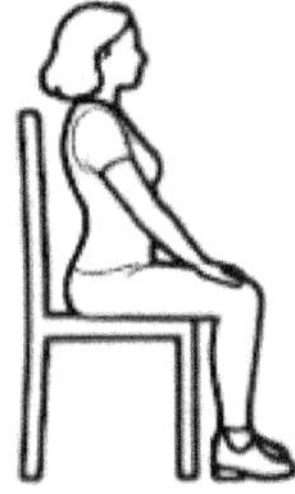 by engaging your abdominal muscles and then relaxing them, promoting a smooth, controlled movement. This movement significantly boosts lumbar flexibility, easing tension and discomfort. Long drives used to be a significant source of discomfort for me, however I've discovered that performing adapted pelvic tilts while seated in my car makes these journeys much more bearable. This simple adjustment has been crucial in introducing mobility to my lower back, effectively reducing discomfort.

When exercising with back pain, it's important to adapt your routine to accommodate your needs and limitations. Maintain a neutral spine during exercises, keeping your back straight and avoiding excessive arching or bending.This alignment supports your spine and reduces stress on the muscles and joints, preventing further pain. Listening to your body and adjusting exercises as needed is crucial for a safe and effective workout.

Proper Posture plays a significant role in back health, both during exercise and in daily activities. One of my primary duties as a personal trainer is ensuring the movements and alignment are on point. Maintaining alignment helps distribute weight evenly across your body, reducing strain on your spine. Simple techniques can help you maintain proper Posture throughout the day. When sitting, ensure your feet are flat on the floor, and your back is supported by a chair. It's very important to relax your shoulders and try to avoid crossing your legs for extended periods. When standing, make sure to distribute your weight evenly, keep your knees slightly bent and your Core engaged. These minor adjustments can make a big difference, alleviating back pain and promoting overall well-being.

Exercises to Enhance Posture

Posture is a fundamental part of your overall health and mobility. Picture your spine as the central pillar of your body, supporting everything from your head to your hips. When your Posture aligns well, this pillar stands strong and straight, reducing the strain on your muscles and joints. It keeps your body balanced, distributes weight evenly, and prevents unnecessary wear and tear. Proper spinal alignment helps maintain the natural curve of your spine, which is crucial for avoiding discomfort and injury.

Furthermore, good Posture positively impacts your breathing and circulation. When you stand or sit with your back straight, your lungs have more room to expand fully, enabling you to take deeper, more efficient breaths. This increased oxygen intake boosts circulation, energizing your body and improving overall vitality.

To improve Posture, incorporate simple exercises into your routine that focus on strengthening the muscles of your back and shoulders. Shoulder blade squeezes are a great start. Stand or sit with your back straight and your arms by your sides. Squeeze your shoulder blades together and hold for a few seconds. Remember to take deep breaths during each exercise. Many of my clients have a tendency to hold their breath throughout an exercise or stretch, but proper breathing will help you achieve the best results. This exercise strengthens the upper back muscles, promoting better Posture.

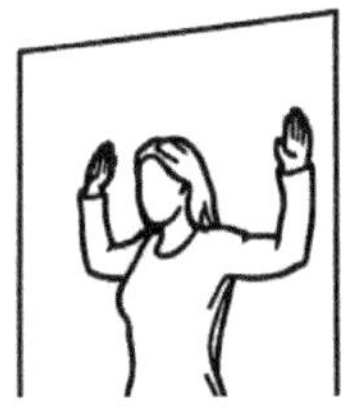 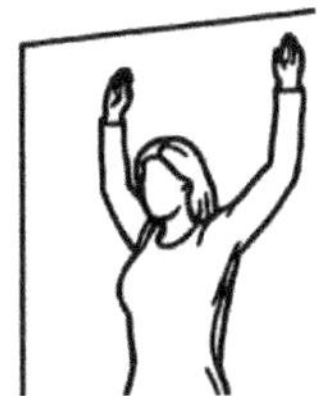

Another effective exercise is wall angels. Stand with your back against a wall, your feet a few inches away. Press your lower back, shoulders, and head against the wall. Slowly raise your arms over your head, making sure to keep your back, head, and arms in contact with the wall. As you lift your arms, keep the elbows and wrists touching the wall as much as possible. If you can't keep your arms fully against the wall, only go as high as possible; however, maintain contact with the wall at all times. From here, slowly extend your arms upward to form a "Y" shape, again while keeping your arms against the wall. Finally, return to the starting position. This movement enhances shoulder flexibility and is an asset to maintaining good Posture.

Maintaining proper Posture throughout the day requires mindfulness and minor adjustments. Set reminders to check your Posture periodically, especially if you spend long hours sitting at a desk or engaged in activities that encourage slouching. Consider ergonomic adjustments to your home and work environments. Ensure your chair offers adequate support and your computer screen is at eye level to reduce neck strain. Simple changes like these can significantly affect how you feel and function daily. The psychological benefits of good Posture are equally important. When you stand tall, you project confidence to the world and yourself. This increased self-esteem can improve your mood and outlook on life, reducing feelings of fatigue and stress. Good Posture encourages a sense of empowerment, reminding you of your strength and resilience. It can transform how you perceive and interact with the world, fostering a positive mental state that enhances well-being. This newfound confidence can inspire you to engage more fully in social activities and pursue interests with renewed enthusiasm. Integrating posture-improving exercises and strategies into your routine will pave the way for a healthier, more active lifestyle. As you become more aware of your Posture, you'll notice improvements in your physical health and mental and emotional well-being. This transformation offers a glimpse into the interconnected nature of body and mind, highlighting the importance of caring for both.

6

MOTIVATIONAL STRATEGIES AND LONG-TERM HABITS

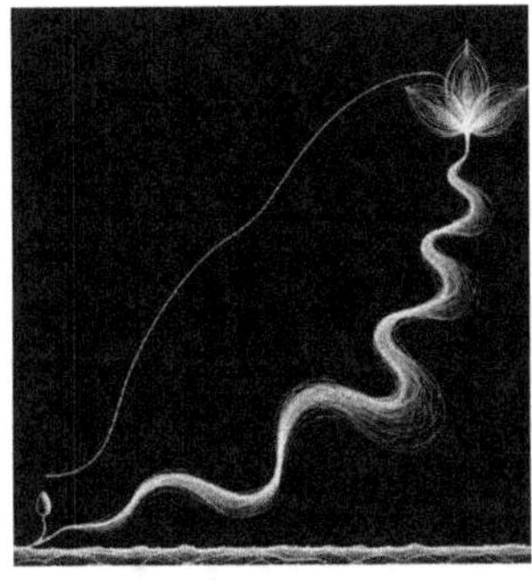

Setting goals isn't just about reaching a destination; it's about giving your efforts direction and infusing your routine with meaning. Whether it's the satisfaction of completing a daily walk or the pride of mastering a new exercise, these milestones transform intent into action, creating a path to sustained progress and fulfillment. The concept of goal-setting takes on a new dimension when we break down long-term aspirations into smaller, manageable steps. Your fitness journey is a series of achievable milestones that lead to more remarkable achievements. Instead of focusing on distant goals that may seem overwhelming, concentrate on incremental progress. For example, if your aim is to improve your balance, start with a simple goal like standing on one leg for a few seconds each day, gradually increasing the duration as your confidence grows. These bite-sized objectives build momentum, each success creating a foundation for the next challenge, and before you know it, you're making strides you once thought impossible.

As discussed in Chapter 1, a structured approach to goal-setting can provide clarity and focus, turning abstract desires into concrete plans. The SMART framework—Specific, Measurable, Achievable, Relevant, and Time-bound—is a tool designed to refine your objectives. For example, a clear and actionable SMART objective would be: "Walk for 10 minutes every day for a week". Measurability allows you to track progress, offering tangible evidence of your efforts. Achievability ensures the goal is within reach, fostering a sense of accomplishment rather than frustration. Relevance aligns the goal with your broader life aspirations, ensuring it holds personal significance. Finally, setting a time-frame instills urgency and discipline, transforming dreams into commitments.

Visualization is a potent ally in maintaining motivation. By picturing your achievements vividly, you reinforce the belief in your potential. A pivotal aspect of my gymnastics career involved mastering the art of visualization. My coaches emphasized the importance of mentally rehearsing each movement and routine, instructing us to practice this technique every night before bed and again each morning. This discipline extended beyond the physical confines of the gym, as I dedicated time daily to visualization. The profound impact this practice had on my success in gymnastics cannot be overstated, underscoring the power of mental preparation in achieving excellence.

Vision boards or journals are practical tools for this practice. Imagine a board adorned with images and words that reflect your goals—perhaps a picture of a serene park where you envision your daily walks or a quote that resonates with your fitness ethos. Journals offer a written reflection, capturing your thoughts, aspirations, and triumphs on paper. Both methods constantly remind you of what you're working towards, instilling a sense of purpose and keeping your motivation alive.

Realistic milestones are the stepping stones to sustained success. Consider increasing your daily step count by just 500 steps, a goal that's both attainable and impactful. It encourages daily movement, subtly enhancing your fitness level without overwhelming you. Another milestone could be completing a balance exercise without support, a testament to your growing strength and stability. These goals are not only reachable but also profoundly satisfying. They demonstrate growth in your abilities, offering tangible proof of your progress. Each milestone achieved boosts your confidence, reinforcing the idea that you are capable of more than you once believed.

Overcoming Exercise Plateaus

Imagine you're on a path, steadily moving forward when suddenly, things seem to stall. This is the essence of an exercise plateau. It's a natural stage in any fitness routine where progress slows, not because of a lack of effort but due to your body adapting to the current level of activity. Our bodies are remarkably efficient; they learn, adjust, and become accustomed to physical demands. When you first start a new exercise regimen, the changes are often noticeable. You might feel stronger and more energized or even see improvements in your strength and balance. However, as your body becomes used to these movements, the same exercises yield lesser results, leading to what seems like stagnation. This adaptation is a double-edged sword; it signifies strength and resilience but can also feel like a roadblock in your fitness progress.

To break through these plateaus, it's crucial to introduce variety and new challenges to your routine. One effective strategy is to change up your exercises. If you've been walking the same route every day, try altering your path or incorporating hills to engage different muscle groups. Interval training can also breathe new life into your routine. By alternating between high and low-intensity periods, you challenge your body in new ways, boosting cardiovascular health and endurance. This variation keeps your muscles guessing and prevents them from settling into a predictable pattern. Incorporating new exercises like cycling or swimming can offer fresh challenges and avoid monotony.

Patience and persistence are essential when facing a plateau. It's easy to feel frustrated when results slow, but progress isn't always linear. Staying committed to your routine, even when it seems futile, is essential. This is the time to set new challenges and goals that are slightly out of reach but achievable with effort. Aim to increase your walking time by a few minutes each week, or try a new strength-training exercise that pushes your limits. These new objectives provide a sense of purpose and direction, helping to maintain motivation even when the going gets tough.

Managing the mental aspects of a plateau is just as important as the physical. Frustration can quickly take over, leaving you feeling defeated. This is where mental resilience techniques come into play. Positive affirmations can shift your mindset, reminding you of your strengths and past accomplishments. Take a moment each day to repeat affirmations like, "I am strong" or "I am capable of change." Meditation practices can also help center your thoughts, provide clarity, and reduce stress. By focusing on your breath and letting go of negative thoughts, you create space for positivity and perseverance. These practices not only enhance your mental well-being but also support your physical goals.

Ultimately, overcoming a plateau requires creativity, commitment, and mental strength. It's about embracing the challenge and seeing it as an opportunity for growth. By varying your routine, setting new goals, and nurturing your mental resilience, you push past stagnation and continue on your path to improved fitness and well-being.

Building a Supportive Community

Imagine setting out on a new endeavor where each step feels a little lighter because you're not alone. In fitness, a supportive community can be this very source of strength. The benefits of having a network are profound. Not only does it provide motivation, but it also fosters accountability. Within a community, experiences are shared, encouragement is abundant, and each member becomes a source of inspiration for the others. When you hear about someone overcoming a similar hurdle, it reinforces the belief that you, too, can achieve your goals. This shared journey creates a bond that enriches every individual's path, turning solitary strides into a collective march toward health and vitality.

Connecting with others might seem daunting, but numerous avenues exist. Local fitness classes or senior groups are excellent starting points. They offer structured environments where individuals with similar goals gather, creating a natural platform for forming connections. The camaraderie in these settings is refreshing, as laughter and shared experiences make each session more than just exercise—it becomes a social event. Online forums and social media groups provide a rich tapestry of support for those who prefer the digital realm. These platforms transcend geographical boundaries, bringing together a diverse array of people striving for better health. Here, you can share tips, celebrate victories, and even discuss challenges, knowing there's a community eager to support you.

Family and friends can play a pivotal role in your fitness pursuits. Encouraging them to join you for family walks or group exercises can transform routine activities into cherished moments of connection. When loved ones participate, the lines between exercise and leisure blur, making fitness an integral part of your lifestyle. They offer more than just companionship; they provide a sense of accountability, motivating you to stick with your routine. Whether it's a weekly walk in the park or a Saturday yoga session, these activities strengthen not only your body but also your relationships. Over time, the shared experience of pursuing health goals can deepen bonds, turning family and friends into your greatest allies on the path to wellness.

Despite the numerous benefits, building a community isn't without its challenges. Physical limitations or mobility issues can make attending in-person events difficult. However, technology offers solutions that bridge these gaps. Virtual meet-ups are an innovative way to connect with others, regardless of physical constraints. Platforms like Zoom or Skype allow you to join group workouts from the comfort of your home. Imagine participating in a virtual fitness class where each participant is connected through screens, sharing the experience in real-time. My husband and I have embarked on a new venture, offering in-home virtual classes. We lead these live sessions, inviting clients of all fitness levels to join us from the comfort of their own homes. These digital connections may not replace face-to-face interactions, but they offer a valuable alternative, ensuring that no one feels isolated in their fitness endeavors.

In this interconnected age, the possibilities for building a supportive community are vast. With a bit of curiosity and willingness, you can find or create a circle that enriches your fitness experience, making each step towards better health a shared triumph.

The Role of Positivity and Motivation

Imagine waking up each day with a sense of enthusiasm and curiosity about what lies ahead. That's the power of a positive mindset. It's not just about feeling good; it's about transforming how you approach challenges and opportunities, particularly in your fitness regimen. When you focus on what you can achieve rather than what stands in your way, exercise becomes more enjoyable and fulfilling. This shift in perspective can make all the difference. Instead of viewing a workout as a daunting task, see it as an opportunity to nurture your body and mind. With this mindset, each step forward becomes a victory, reinforcing your commitment to health and well-being.

Cultivating this positivity starts with small, intentional practices. One effective method is gratitude journaling. Gratitude journaling stands as my favorite method for maintaining a positive outlook, not only in my fitness journey but in all aspects of my life. By taking a few moments each day to jot down what you're thankful for, you help and train your mind to focus on the positive aspects of your life. This simple practice can shift your outlook, making it easier to see the good in every situation. Surrounding yourself with positive and uplifting people also plays a crucial role. Whether it's spending time with cheerful friends, watching inspiring videos, or reading motivational stories, these influences can elevate your mood and reinforce your positive mindset. Choose activities and people that energize you, creating an environment that supports your goals and enhances your happiness.

Motivation is what gets you moving, even on days when you'd rather stay in bed. To sustain motivation, consider incorporating various tools and resources into your routine. Inspirational fitness stories or podcasts can be powerful motivators, offering insights and encouragement from those who have walked a similar path. Listening to others' experiences can reignite your passion and remind you of the benefits of staying active. Motivational quotes or daily affirmations can also serve as gentle nudges, encouraging you to keep going when motivation wanes. Display these reminders in places you'll see them often, like on your fridge or bathroom mirror, ensuring they are part of your daily routine. I maintain a motivational quote as my phone's wallpaper, ensuring it's the first thing I see whenever I use my phone. This serves as my personal nudge, a constant reminder to keep pushing forward.

Amidst the pursuit of goals, it's important to practice self-compassion and kindness. There will be days when things don't go as planned, and setbacks are inevitable. During these times, it's crucial to treat yourself with the same care and understanding you would offer a friend. Recognize that nobody is perfect and that progress often comes with hurdles. Self-care and relaxation techniques can help you navigate these challenges with grace. Whether it's taking a warm bath, enjoying a leisurely walk in nature, or indulging in a favorite hobby, these activities replenish your spirit. Prioritizing self-care ensures that you're not only physically fit but emotionally resilient, equipping you to face whatever comes your way.

Incorporating these practices into your life creates a foundation of positivity and motivation that supports your fitness goals. By embracing an optimistic outlook, surrounding yourself with uplifting influences, and practicing kindness towards yourself, you cultivate an environment where growth and progress thrive. This holistic approach not only enhances your fitness journey but enriches every aspect of your life, making each day more vibrant and fulfilling.

Creating a Personalized Exercise Log

Imagine sitting down after a fulfilling workout, a sense of accomplishment washing over you. There's great value in capturing this moment and in documenting your journey. An exercise log does just that. It's more than just a record of activity; it's a powerful tool to track your progress, providing insights that can fuel your motivation. By logging your workouts, you begin to notice patterns—perhaps you feel more energized on days you exercise in the morning, or maybe specific exercises consistently lift your mood. These insights can help you refine your routine, focusing on what works best for your body and mind.

Setting up a personalized exercise log is a straightforward process, yet one that can have lasting benefits. Start by deciding whether you prefer a digital format or a classic paper journal. Each has its advantages. Digital logs can offer convenience, with apps providing reminders and easy access to data. Paper journals, on the other hand, allow for a tactile experience, letting you physically jot down notes and reflect on your progress. Whichever you choose, structure your log with sections dedicated to your goals, achievements, and reflections. This organization helps you keep track of what you're working towards, what you've accomplished, and what thoughts or feelings arise during your workouts.

To make your log comprehensive, consider what elements you might include. Documenting the duration and type of exercise is a good start. Did you walk for 30 minutes today or perhaps engage in balance exercises? Note these details. Also, capture your mood and energy levels before and after workouts. You might find that certain activities consistently boost your spirits or help you unwind. This information not only provides a record of your physical activity but also paints a picture of how your routine impacts your overall well-being. By observing these patterns, you can make informed decisions and adjust your routine to maximize benefits.

Follow the QR link from Chapter 1 to access a bonus log journal in full color and start tracking your progress with a planner I have created that tracks not only the exercises but also other factors that impact our physical health.

Reflection is a vital component of your exercise log. At the end of each week, take some time to review your entries. Consider what went well and where there might be room for improvement. This regular reflection fosters a deeper understanding of your personal growth. You might notice that your endurance has increased, or perhaps you've become more flexible. These observations can enhance your motivation, reminding you of the progress you've made and the potential for further development. Writing an end-of-week summary can provide clarity, allowing you to set new intentions for the week ahead. This process turns your exercise log into a dynamic tool for self-discovery and improvement, guiding you on a path of continuous growth.

Celebrating Small Victories

In life's vast landscape, where goals and milestones often seem distant, it's the small victories that illuminate our path. Recognizing these achievements, no matter how minor they may appear, is crucial for maintaining motivation and reinforcing positive behavior. Each accomplishment, whether it's taking an extra step or completing a full set of exercises, is a testament to your commitment and perseverance. When you acknowledge these moments, you validate your efforts, turning each one into a building block for greater success. This recognition fosters a mindset of progress, where every small step forward becomes a powerful affirmation of your dedication to health and well-being.

Celebrating these milestones can take many forms, each as unique as the individual. Treating yourself to a favorite activity or hobby is one way to honor your progress. Whether it's an afternoon spent immersed in a good book or a leisurely stroll through a park, these moments of joy are rewards in themselves. Sharing your achievements with friends or family can also amplify the pleasure of success. When you tell a loved one about a new personal best or an exercise you finally mastered, their encouragement and pride can be incredibly uplifting. These celebrations create a sense of community, where your victories are shared and cherished, enhancing your motivation to continue striving for more.

The emotional benefits of recognizing progress extend beyond the immediate pleasure of celebration. Each acknowledgment of achievement boosts self-esteem and happiness, reinforcing a sense of accomplishment and pride. This positive feedback loop strengthens your resolve, making it easier to face new challenges. When you celebrate your progress, you're not just marking a point in time; you're building a mental reservoir of confidence and resilience. This confidence spills over into other areas of life, encouraging you to take on new endeavors with the belief that you can succeed. As your self-esteem grows, so does your capacity to embrace change and pursue dreams with vigor.

To maintain this positive trajectory, establishing a reward system for forthcoming goals can be highly beneficial. This strategy is one I often employ to align my progress and motivation. By orchestrating mini-celebrations upon achieving certain milestones, we honor the dedication behind our efforts. These rewards, while not lavish, act as poignant acknowledgments of our perseverance. Personally, rewarding myself with fresh gym attire or a day at the spa stands as my way of commemorating these achievements. The anticipation of these rewards adds an element of excitement to your efforts, transforming each milestone into a stepping stone toward personal growth. This approach not only motivates continued effort but also turns the journey of fitness into a series of joyful experiences.

As you celebrate your small victories, remember that each one is a testament to your journey and growth. They are the threads that weave together the tapestry of your fitness experience, creating a rich and vibrant picture of progress and achievement. By embracing these moments of triumph, you cultivate a mindset of gratitude and positivity, setting the stage for future success.

7

EXERCISES FOR EVERYDAY INDEPENDENCE

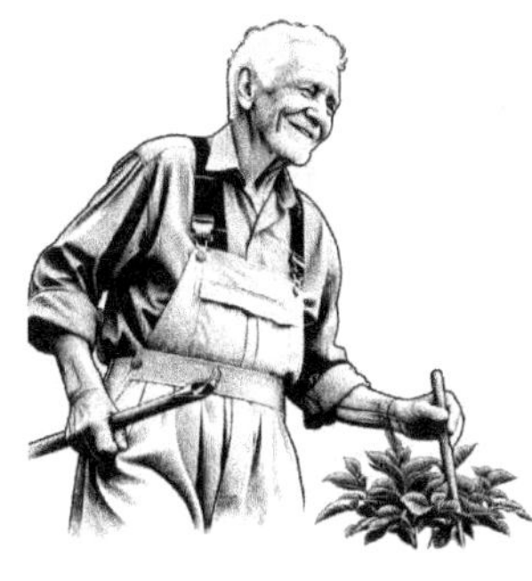

Imagine waking up each morning with the confidence that you can handle whatever the day brings. Whether it's reaching for a mug on a high shelf or getting up from your favorite chair, these everyday actions are made easier with functional fitness. Functional fitness is about strengthening the movements you perform daily. This type of fitness focuses on the practical applications of exercise, ensuring your body is prepared for real-life activities. It's about enhancing the muscles you use in routine tasks like lifting groceries or climbing stairs, making them smoother and safer. By integrating these exercises into your life, you will gain more independence and improve your quality of life.

Functional fitness is about mimicking the activities that fill your day. Picture yourself squatting to pick up a dropped pen or reaching to dust the top shelf. These movements are exercises in disguise and form the basis of functional fitness. Squats, for instance, are not just for the gym. They're the motions you engage in when sitting in or standing from a chair. Practicing squats strengthens your legs and core, providing stability and making these transitions effortless. Reaching exercises, on the other hand, prepare you for tasks like retrieving items from high places. By stretching your arms and engaging your core, you improve your range of motion and reduce the risk of straining. These exercises are simple, yet they empower you to handle daily activities with ease.

The benefits of functional fitness extend beyond physical strength. By improving your functional fitness, you enhance your overall energy levels, making everyday tasks feel less taxing. This energy boost means more time and enthusiasm for the activities you love, whether gardening, playing with grandchildren, or enjoying a leisurely walk. The risk of injury also decreases as your body becomes more resilient and capable of handling the demands of daily life without strain. This resilience translates into confidence, knowing that you can move through your day with assurance and grace. Functional fitness is not just about exercise; it's a way to enrich your life, making each day more enjoyable and fulfilling.

Integrating these exercises into your daily routine can be seamless. Consider performing squats while brushing your teeth. This not only strengthens your muscles but also makes the most of your time, turning mundane moments into opportunities for fitness. While watching television, practice reaching exercises during commercial breaks. Stand up, stretch your arms towards the ceiling, and engage your core as if reaching for an invisible item. These minor adjustments transform everyday moments into steps toward better health. By incorporating functional fitness exercises into your routine, you create a lifestyle that supports your independence and well-being.

Enhancing Strength with Simple Movements

As the years go by, maintaining muscle strength becomes a cornerstone of health and vitality. It's about more than just being able to lift heavy objects or perform strenuous activities; it's about preserving the muscle mass that naturally diminishes with age. This strength is crucial for balance and coordination, two essential components that enable you to move confidently. When muscles are strong, they support your joints, making everyday movements safer and more efficient. Engaging in regular strength training helps to counteract the muscle loss associated with aging, ensuring that you can continue to enjoy the activities you love without hesitation.

To build strength without the need for complex equipment, consider incorporating simple exercises into your daily routine.

As seen in Chapter 1 and Chapter 3, Wall push-ups are an excellent way to enhance upper body strength. For lower body strength, seated leg extensions are a practical choice.

This movement strengthens the quadriceps, supporting the knees and improving overall leg stability.

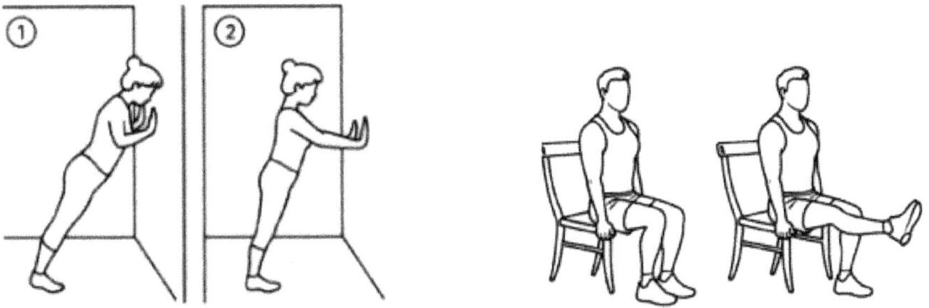

Progressive overload is an important aspect of continuing strength gains. Start with a manageable number of repetitions, and as your body adapts, gradually increase the challenge. You can add resistance using household items like water bottles, which act as makeshift weights. As you become stronger, increase the number of repetitions or sets, pushing your muscles to new limits. This gradual increase encourages muscle growth and adaptation, ensuring that your strength continues to build over time. Remember, the goal is steady progress, allowing your body to effectively respond to increased demands.

Safety should always be your priority when engaging in strength training. Proper form and correct alignment are crucial to prevent injury. Focus on maintaining a neutral spine, engaging your core, and avoiding any jerky movements. Take time to warm up before starting your exercises, perhaps by marching in place or doing shoulder rolls. These activities prepare your muscles and joints, reducing the risk of strains. After your workout, a cool-down period with gentle stretching helps to ease your muscles back into a resting state, preventing stiffness and promoting recovery.

Strength training doesn't have to be complex or intimidating. With these simple exercises and safety guidelines, you can effectively build and maintain muscle strength from the comfort of your home. By prioritizing strength training, you invest in your health and independence, empowering yourself to live an active and fulfilling life.

Balance Techniques for Outdoor Activities

Stepping outside offers more than just a change of scenery; it provides an opportunity to engage in activities that enhance balance and stability. Improved balance is crucial for safely navigating the uneven terrains often encountered outdoors. Whether you're walking on a gravel path or hiking up a gentle hill, having stable footing reduces the risk of falls and injuries. This confidence extends to enjoying hobbies such as gardening, where you might find yourself bending, reaching, and stepping over obstacles. The ability to move securely on varied surfaces not only enhances your outdoor experience but also encourages a more active lifestyle.

To improve your balance outdoors, consider incorporating exercises that adapt to the natural environment. Walking on different surfaces, such as grass or sand, requires different muscle engagements, helping to strengthen your stabilizer muscles, which are necessary for balance. One of the initial rehabilitative exercises recommended to me following a gymnastics-induced ankle fracture involved walking on grass. The natural unevenness of the terrain engaged and strengthened various stabilizer muscles throughout my lower body, providing a gentle yet effective method to regain balance and coordination. This activity not only aided my physical recovery but also reacquainted my body with the subtle shifts required to maintain stability on variable surfaces. Another effective exercise is stepping over obstacles. Find a safe area with small, manageable obstacles like stones or logs, and practice stepping over them with deliberate, controlled movements. This enhances your agility and improves your ability to handle unexpected changes in your path, making outdoor adventures safer and more enjoyable.

Safety should always be at the forefront when exercising outside. Selecting the right footwear is crucial; choose shoes with good support and non-slip soles to provide stability. Be mindful of the weather conditions as well. A sunny day might be inviting, but extreme heat can quickly lead to exhaustion, while rain can make surfaces slippery. Always check the forecast before heading out and dress appropriately for the conditions. Consider carrying a walking stick for additional support on uneven paths. This not only aids balance but also provides an extra point of contact with the ground, increasing your stability. These precautions help ensure that your outdoor activities are both safe and beneficial.

Exercising in nature offers a unique array of benefits that go beyond physical fitness. The serene environment of a park or garden can significantly enhance your mood, reducing stress and promoting relaxation. The gentle rustle of leaves, the sound of birds, and the feeling of the sun on your skin contribute to a sense of well-being and tranquility. While engaging in outdoor exercises, you have the unique opportunity to incorporate grounding techniques alongside your physical activities, enhancing the overall experience. Grounding involves direct contact with Mother Nature, promoting physiological and electrophysiological changes that contribute to your well-being. As you perform balance and agility exercises on natural surfaces like grass or sand, take a moment to connect with the earth beneath your feet. Feel the texture of the ground, feel the coolness or the warmth that it brings. This connection not only enhances your balance training by providing a variable and challenging terrain but also helps to center your mind, reduce stress, and improve your mood. Additionally, spending time outdoors increases your exposure to vitamin D, which is essential for bone health and immune function. This exposure, combined with physical activity, creates a holistic approach to health, nurturing both body and mind. The simple act of moving outside can transform your exercise routine into a refreshing and invigorating experience.

Outdoor balance exercises are not just about building physical strength; they are about reconnecting with nature and yourself. They offer a break from the confines of indoor routines, encouraging you to explore and enjoy the world around you. The fresh air, natural beauty, and varied terrains provide endless opportunities for movement and growth. As you practice these exercises, you'll find that each step taken outdoors is a step towards improved health and happiness.

Exercises to Improve Gait and Stability

Gait is a term that encompasses the way you walk, and it plays a pivotal role in your mobility. It's more than just putting one foot in front of the other; gait involves the coordination of your entire body, which impacts your ability to move with ease and confidence. A stable and confident gait is a cornerstone of independence. It allows you to navigate your environment securely, whether you're strolling through your home or venturing out into the community. A strong gait helps prevent falls, a common concern as we age, by providing a steady and predictable movement pattern. When your gait is smooth and controlled, it ensures that each step is deliberate, reducing the risk of trips or missteps. This connection between gait and fall prevention underscores its importance in maintaining mobility, allowing you to live your life without unnecessary limitations.

There are specific exercises that can be incorporated into your routine to enhance your gait. Heel-to-toe walking is a simple yet effective exercise that can improve your stride. To perform this, walk in a straight line, placing the heel of your front foot directly against the toes of your back foot with each step. This exercise not only strengthens the muscles in your legs but also trains your body to maintain balance, promoting a more stable walk. Another beneficial exercise is high knees, which involves lifting each knee toward your chest alternately while walking in place. This movement strengthens the leg muscles, particularly the thighs, and enhances balance by engaging the core. Both exercises are straightforward and can be performed almost anywhere, making them easy to integrate into your daily activities.

Assessing your gait is an important step in understanding your mobility and making improvements where necessary. One effective method is to use video recordings. Set up a camera or ask someone to record you as you walk naturally. Review the footage to observe your posture, stride length, and any imbalances. This self-assessment can provide valuable insights into areas needing improvement. Additionally, seeking feedback from healthcare professionals can offer expert guidance tailored to your specific needs. They can help identify subtle issues that may not be apparent during self-assessment, providing exercises and strategies to enhance your gait further.

Posture plays a crucial role in maintaining a healthy gait. The correct alignment of the head, shoulders, and hips ensures that your body moves efficiently and reduces strain on muscles and joints. Picture an imaginary line running from the top of your head through your spine to your feet. This alignment helps distribute your body weight evenly, minimizing the risk of injury and enhancing your balance. To maintain this posture while walking, focus on keeping your shoulders relaxed and your head up, with your gaze forward rather than down. Engage your core muscles to support your spine, and let your arms swing naturally by your sides. These simple techniques can make a significant difference in the quality of your gait, contributing to improved mobility and overall well-being.

Integrating Routines into Morning Rituals

Each morning offers a fresh start, a chance to set the tone for the day ahead. Incorporating exercise into your morning routine awakens your body, invigorates your senses and sharpens your focus. A morning workout boosts your energy levels, giving you that extra pep in your step and enhancing alertness. This heightened state of awareness not only helps you tackle your daily tasks but also establishes a positive and proactive mindset. It's a simple yet powerful way to begin the day on a high note, ready to face whatever comes your way with enthusiasm and clarity.

Consider starting your day with a few simple stretches as you rise. These movements gently coax your muscles into action, relieving any stiffness from the night. Imagine reaching up towards the ceiling, lengthening your spine, and feeling a gentle stretch through your sides. This act not only eases tension but also promotes circulation, waking up your body from head to toe. Following your stretches, a morning walk can do wonders for your metabolism. Whether it's a brisk walk around the block or a leisurely stroll through your neighborhood, this activity stimulates your cardiovascular system and kickstarts calorie burning.

Fitting these routines into a busy schedule may seem challenging, but with a few practical adjustments, it's entirely achievable. Setting a consistent wake-up time works wonders; it establishes a regular rhythm for your body, making it easier to start the day active and ready. An effective strategy I've adopted is to prepare my workout clothes the night before. This simple step eliminates any hesitation in the morning, letting me focus entirely on my exercise routine. Organizing your morning this way smooths the transition into your daily tasks, effortlessly weaving physical activity into the fabric of everyday life.

Consistency is crucial in forming a morning exercise habit. By incorporating exercise into your morning ritual, you create a habit loop—a cycle that reinforces itself with each repetition. As you repeat these exercises daily, they become a natural part of your routine, something you look forward to rather than an obligation. Seeing your improvements over time, whether it's increased energy or a more positive outlook, can provide the encouragement needed to continue. This sense of accomplishment fuels your desire to maintain these practices, reinforcing the positive impact they have on your life.

Evening Exercises for Relaxation

While I thrive on the energizing benefits of exercising in the morning, the tranquility of the evening offers a perfect backdrop for unwinding, allowing both the mind and body to release the stresses of the day and ease into a state of relaxation. As daylight fades, it signals our bodies to transition from the day's hustle to the peaceful embrace of the night. Incorporating gentle exercises during this time can significantly enhance this transition, facilitating a reduction in stress and a promotion of relaxation, thereby preparing us for a night of restorative sleep. This approach not only soothes the nervous system but also sets the stage for a deep and peaceful slumber.

Consider incorporating calming exercises into your evening routine. Gentle yoga poses, such as the child's pose or the seated forward bend, are excellent for releasing tension and promoting relaxation. These poses encourage your muscles to relax and your mind to settle, creating a sense of peace and tranquility. As you move through each pose, focus on your breathing, inhaling deeply and exhaling slowly. This mindful breathing enhances the relaxation effect, helping you to let go of the day's stress. Meditation is another powerful tool you can use. Find a comfortable seated position, close your eyes, and concentrate on your breath. Allow any lingering thoughts from the day to drift away, leaving you with a sense of calm and clarity.

Creating a calming environment for your evening exercises enhances their effectiveness. Dim the lights to signal to your body that it's time to relax. Low lighting helps to reduce stimulation, encouraging your mind to slow down. Soft, calming music can also be beneficial, providing a soothing background that complements your movements and breathing. Consider adding aromatherapy to your routine. Scents like lavender or chamomile are known for their relaxing properties.

The transition from activity to rest is an important part of your evening routine. Establish a pre-sleep routine that includes a set time for your exercises, followed by activities that promote relaxation, such as reading a book or taking a warm bath. This routine acts as a signal to your body that it's time to prepare for sleep, helping to create a smooth transition from the busyness of the day to the calm of night. It's also important to avoid screens and stimulants before bed. The blue light emitted by screens can interfere with your body's natural sleep cycle, making it harder to fall asleep. Instead, choose activities that encourage relaxation, setting the stage for a restful night's sleep. As you embrace these practices, you nurture your well-being, ensuring that each day ends in peace and tranquility.

8

ADVANCED TECHNIQUES FOR IMPROVED STABILITY

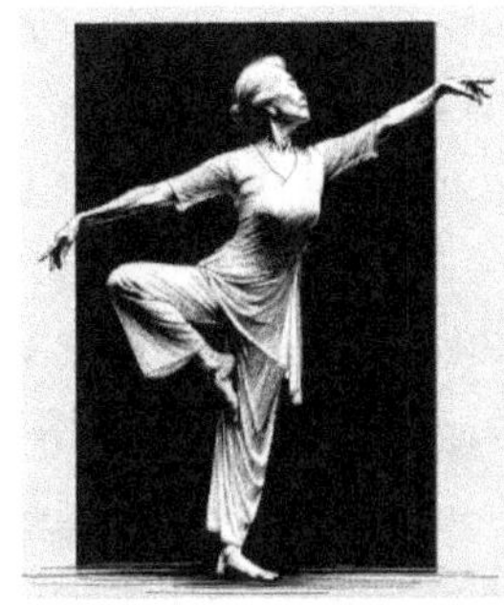

Imagine standing on one leg, much like a flamingo, poised and balanced. This simple act can unlock a world of stability and strength within you. One-legged stands might seem challenging at first, but they offer profound benefits that extend far beyond the exercise itself. By mastering this skill, you'll not only enhance your balance but also strengthen the core muscles that support your everyday movements. One-legged stands are a testament to the power of simplicity in achieving complex improvements in your physical health.

The benefits of one-legged stands are multifaceted. They work wonders for your proprioception, which is your body's ability to sense its position in space. Proprioception strengthens your awareness and control over your movements, making you more adept at navigating your environment with confidence. Furthermore, these stands are excellent for fortifying your ankles and knees, which are crucial for maintaining stability. When you engage in this exercise, you activate and strengthen the muscles around these joints, providing a solid foundation for balance and agility. This exercise can serve as a cornerstone in your fitness routine, offering both immediate and long-term benefits to your physical health.

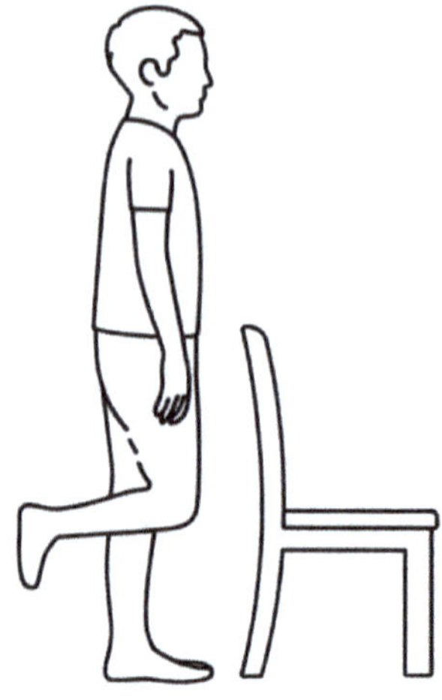

Starting with one-legged stands requires a clear strategy and patience. Begin by standing near a wall or chair for support, ensuring your safety as you practice. Place your feet hip-width apart, and slowly lift one foot off the ground. Focus on a point in front of you to help maintain your balance. This technique, which I've honed from my decade as a gymnast, involves focusing on a single point in the distance. This method is particularly effective during exercises that involve spinning, as it helps to prevent dizziness by giving the brain a stable reference point.

Similarly, when engaging in balance-focused exercises, this focal point technique is invaluable. It helps to maintain stability by anchoring your concentration, allowing for a more controlled and steady posture. This simple but powerful strategy enhances your ability to perform exercises with precision, contributing significantly to your overall balance and coordination. Hold this position for a few seconds, gradually increasing the duration as you become more stable. It's important to keep your core engaged and maintain a straight posture, as this will aid in balance and prevent strain. As you practice, aim to extend the time you can hold the pose, challenging yourself a little more each day. This gradual progression not only builds physical strength but also boosts your confidence in your abilities.

Safety is paramount when practicing one-legged stands. Always perform this exercise on a stable surface, free from any potential hazards. Having a support nearby, like a sturdy chair or wall, provides reassurance and allows you to focus on the exercise without fear of falling. Wear comfortable, supportive footwear to enhance stability and reduce the risk of slipping. As with any exercise, listen to your body's signals. If you feel discomfort or instability, take a moment to rest and readjust. Safety should always be your top priority, ensuring a positive and productive exercise experience.

To keep things fresh and challenging, consider incorporating progression techniques into your practice. Once you feel comfortable with the basic stand, try closing your eyes. This reduces your reliance on visual cues, enhancing your balance and proprioceptive abilities. For an added challenge, hold a lightweight object in your hands. This requires increased focus and control, further engaging your core and improving your balance. These incremental challenges not only make the exercise more engaging but also lead to greater improvements in your stability and strength.

Improved agility also plays a crucial role in daily life. It allows you to react quickly when navigating obstacles, such as stepping over a curb or moving through a crowded area. As our reflexes naturally slow with age, maintaining agility becomes even more important. Agility helps prevent falls and injuries by enabling you to adjust your footing quickly and efficiently. Moreover, it enhances overall movement efficiency, allowing you to conserve energy and move with less effort.

As previously mentioned in Chapter 2, safety is paramount, especially when progressing to a more advanced version of the exercise. To ensure safe practice while performing dynamic movements, it's important to take a few precautions. First, always choose a clear space free of obstacles. This not only reduces the risk of tripping but also allows you to focus fully on the exercise. Wearing appropriate footwear is equally important. Select shoes with good support and non-slip soles to provide stability and minimize the risk of slipping. As you begin, start slowly to familiarize yourself with the movements, gradually increasing speed as you gain confidence. It's essential to listen to your body and rest if you feel any discomfort. Safety should always be your priority, ensuring a positive and productive workout experience.

By incorporating some of the exercises demonstrated throughout the following pages, it will foster a sense of control over your movements, building confidence as you progress and will strengthen both body and mind. They challenge your coordination, improve your agility, and enhance your ability to navigate life's unpredictability with grace and assurance. As you practice, you'll notice that these exercises bring a sense of vitality and energy, invigorating your daily activities and empowering you to live with greater freedom and independence.

** Progression for Standing Marches **

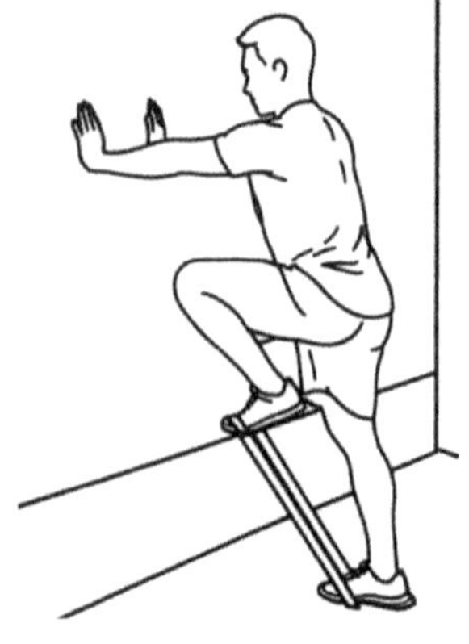

Adding resistance bands to standing marches increases the challenge, enhancing lower-body strength, coordination, and stability while engaging additional muscle groups. Here's how to progress the exercise with resistance bands. Use a looped resistance band or tie a long band into a loop. Select a band with light to medium resistance, ensuring you can maintain proper form throughout the exercise.

Progression Steps

1.Start with Band at Ankles

- Place the resistance band around both feet.

- Stand tall with feet hip-width apart, ensuring the band is taut but not overly stretched.

- Lift one knee toward your chest against the band's resistance, then lower it back down. Alternate legs.

- Hold on to a surface for additional stability.

- Focus on slow, controlled movements to prevent the band from snapping back.

2. Move Band to Above Knees

- Position the band just above your knees to target your hip flexors and thighs more directly.

- March in place, lifting each knee as high as is comfortable while maintaining balance and proper posture.

- Once you feel comfortable without the additional stability of a wall, you can try the movement standing in place near a support should you need.

3. Incorporate Arm Movements
- For additional difficulty, add a natural arm swing or hold light weights in your hands to increase cardiovascular effort and upper-body engagement.

- Ensure the arms and legs move in a coordinated rhythm to enhance coordination.

4. March Forward and Backward
- Once you are able to master the previous steps, try stepping forward with each march, ensuring the band's tension remains steady.

- Reverse the motion, marching backward, which engages stabilizing muscles and challenges your coordination further.

5. Single-Leg March Hold
- Increasing the difficulty even more, lift one knee and hold it in position for 3–5 seconds before lowering it back down.

- Alternate legs, focusing on balance and engaging your core to prevent swaying.

6. Increase Band Resistance
- Gradually switch to a band with higher resistance as your strength and coordination improve.

Benefits of These Progressions

These progressions are excellent for strengthening the hip flexors, thighs, and calves, building lower body strength while enhancing joint stability and balance. It also improves coordination by requiring controlled movements and contributes to cardiovascular endurance by increasing heart rate. Together, these benefits make it a valuable addition to a fitness routine focused on functional strength and overall mobility.

** Progression for Seated Leg Extensions **

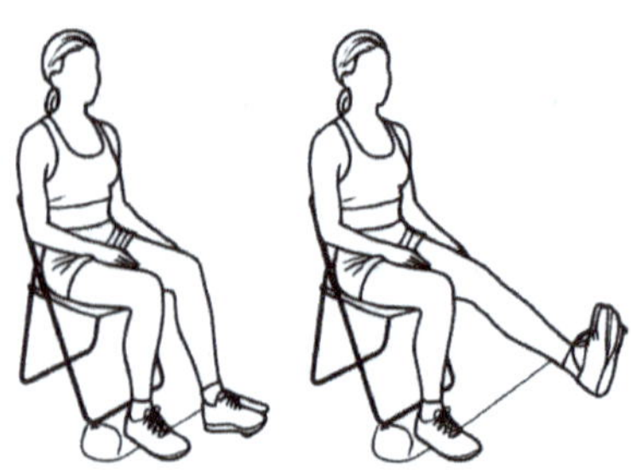

The gradual progressions from single leg extension below allow for safe improvement in lower-body strength, knee stability, and balance. Adding resistance bands to seated leg extensions increases the challenge by further strengthening the quadriceps and engaging additional muscle groups, while improving overall leg stability and control.

Progression Steps

1. Double-Leg Extensions

- Keep the band around your ankles or above your knees, depending on your strength level.

- Simultaneously extend both legs straight out in front of you.

- Hold for 2–3 seconds at the top of the movement, then lower both legs back to the starting position.

2. Add a Hold

- While performing single-leg or double-leg extensions, hold the extended position for 3–5 seconds.

- Focus on maintaining tension in your quadriceps and preventing your back from slouching.

- Gradually increase the hold duration as your strength improves.

3. Incorporate Core Engagement

- Sit slightly away from the backrest of the chair to activate your core.

- Perform leg extensions while maintaining an upright posture and engaging your abdominal muscles to prevent swaying.

- To increase difficulty, extend both legs simultaneously while keeping your core engaged.

4. Increase Resistance

- Switch to a band with higher resistance as your strength improves.

- Start with fewer repetitions (6–8) to adapt to the increased tension, then work up to 12–15 reps.

5. Elevated Seated Position or Standing

- Sit on a slightly higher surface, such as a workout bench, so your legs hang freely.

- If you chose to stand, secure yourself by standing or leaning on a sturdy surface.

- Perform single leg extensions with a full range of motion, ensuring your quads engage throughout.

Benefits of These Progressions

Progressing leg extensions gradually strengthens the quadriceps and core, which in turn improves knee stability and joint mobility. These progressions also support the safe development of balance and coordination, leading to better control and movement efficiency. As strength increases, the risk of injury decreases, allowing for enhanced overall leg function and stability fostering confidence, strength, and functional mobility for everyday activities.

** Progressions for Shoulder Circles **

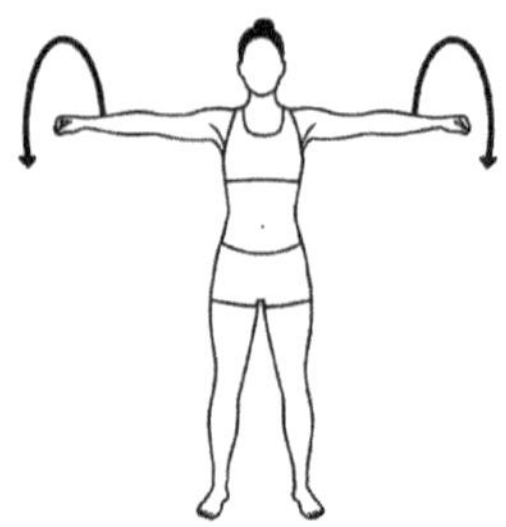

Progressing from seated shoulder circles, standing shoulder circles engage the core and lower body to promote full-body coordination which helps to strengthen the upper body, improve shoulder flexibility, and enhance overall coordination, supporting better posture and ease of movement in daily tasks.

Progression Steps

1. Basic Arm Circles Without Resistance

- Sit on a sturdy chair with your back straight and feet flat on the ground.

- Extend your arms out to the sides at shoulder height, palms facing down.

- Perform small circular motions forward for 10–15 seconds, then reverse direction.

- Focus on keeping your arms level and engaging your shoulder muscles.

2. Add Light Resistance Bands

- Hold a light resistance band between your hands with arms extended out to the sides.

- Perform small forward arm circles while keeping tension in the band.

- Ensure your shoulder blades stay down and back throughout the movement.

3. Increase Circle Size

- Perform larger, controlled arm circles while holding the resistance band taut.

- Move through a greater range of motion, maintaining shoulder stability and core engagement.

4. Add an Isometric Hold
   - After completing each set of arm circles, hold your arms extended outward with the band under tension for 10–15 seconds.

   - Focus on maintaining shoulder and arm alignment during the hold.

   - Gradually increase the duration of the hold as your strength improves.

5. Incorporate Core Engagement
   - Sit slightly away from the backrest to activate your core and improve posture.

   - Perform arm circles while maintaining an upright, stable torso.

   - This engages the core muscles, enhancing overall stability and reducing compensatory movements.

6. Progress to Standing Arm Circles
   - Transition to a standing position for improved stability and balance training.

   - Perform arm circles as before, focusing on maintaining a strong, upright posture.

Benefits of These Progressions

These exercise progression builds shoulder strength, particularly in the rotator cuff and upper back muscles, while improving shoulder stability and reinforcing proper shoulder alignment and spinal posture. It engages stabilizing muscles in the shoulders, upper back, and core, contributing to better posture and overall stability, which are essential for maintaining balance. Incorporating this progression several times a week will help build strength, endurance, and control in the shoulder region, ensuring steady and safe improvement.

** Progression for Shoulder Press **

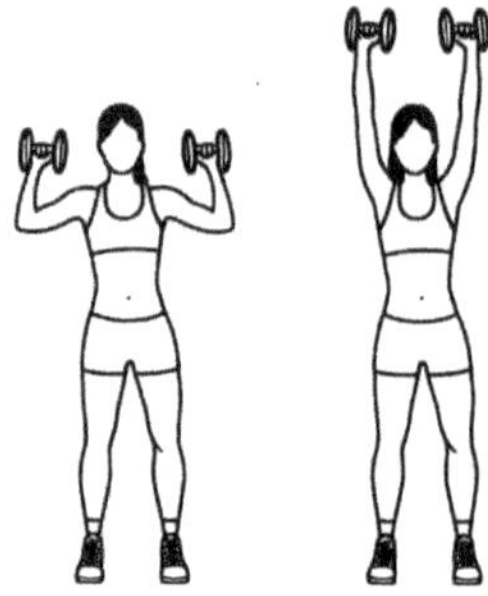

Progressing from seated shoulder presses, standing shoulder presses engage the core and lower body, promoting full-body strength and coordination. This movement builds upper-body strength, enhances shoulder stability, and supports better posture and functional mobility in everyday activities.

Progression Steps

1. Basic Seated Shoulder Press Without Resistance

- Sit on a sturdy chair with your back straight and feet flat on the ground.

- Hold your arms at shoulder height, elbows bent at 90 degrees, and palms facing forward.

- Slowly press your hands upward until your arms are fully extended overhead.

- Lower your hands back to the starting position with control.

2. Add Light Resistance Bands or Dumbbells

- Hold a light resistance band anchored under your chair or light dumbbells in your hands.

- Perform the same pressing motion, focusing on controlled movements and steady breathing.

- Ensure your core remains engaged to support proper posture.

3. Transition to Standing Shoulder Press Without Resistance

- Stand with your feet hip-width apart, maintaining an upright posture.

- Perform the pressing motion without resistance, focusing on shoulder stability.

- Engage your core and avoid arching your lower back.

4. Incorporate Light Resistance in a Standing Position

- Use a resistance band anchored under your feet or light dumbbells.

- Perform standing shoulder presses with slow, deliberate movements.

- Keep your core tight to prevent excessive movement in the torso.

5. Increase Resistance Gradually

- Switch to a heavier resistance band or heavier dumbbells as your strength improves.

- Perform fewer repetitions (6–8) initially, then increase to 10–12 reps as you adapt.

- Ensure movements remain controlled and precise, even with increased resistance.

6. Add an Overhead Hold

- After completing each set, hold the dumbbells or resistance band in the extended overhead position for 10–15 seconds.

- Maintain steady breathing and focus on shoulder stability and core engagement.

- Gradually increase the duration of the hold as your strength builds.

Benefits of These Progressions

Incorporating exercises that target full upper body strength, particularly the shoulders, upper back, and triceps, enhances shoulder stability and reduces the risk of injury. These exercises, when performed regularly several times a week, contribute to steady and safe improvement in strength, endurance, and shoulder control. Over time, this progression helps build confidence, functional capability, and overall upper body stability, ensuring long-term benefits for your fitness routine.

** Progression for Modified Push-Ups **

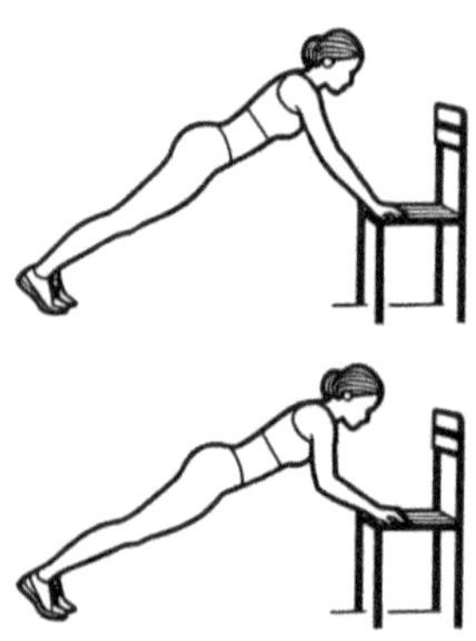

Progressing from basic wall push-ups to more advanced variations enhances upper body strength, engages core muscles, and promotes full-body coordination. This progression strengthens the chest, shoulders, and arms while improving posture and functional movement.

Progression Steps

1. Basic Wall Push-Up
   - Start with an upright position to develop foundational upper body strength.

   - Focus on engaging your core and maintaining a straight line from head to heels.

2. Step Back for Increased Resistance
   - Moving your feet farther from the wall increases the difficulty by adding resistance.

   - Inhale as you lower yourself towards the wall, and exhale as you push back up.

3. Single-Leg Wall Push-Up
   - Lifting one leg shifts weight distribution, enhancing core and stabilizer engagement. Step one foot off the ground and lift it behind you, balancing on the other leg. Keep your body straight, engaging your core and maintaining a neutral spine.

   - Inhale as you lower yourself towards the wall, and exhale as you push back up.

4. Incline Push-Up on a Sturdy Surface
   - Place a sturdy chair against a wall or a stable surface to prevent it from sliding.

Ensure the seat is at a height that allows you to perform the push-up comfortably

- Place your hands on the edge of the chair, slightly wider than shoulder-width apart and step your feet back so your body forms a straight line from your head to your heels. Keep your core engaged and avoid letting your hips sag or your back arch.

- Bend your elbows and lower your chest toward the chair in a controlled manner. Keep your elbows at a 45-degree angle from your body, not flaring out too wide. Press through your palms to straighten your arms, lifting your chest back up to the starting position. Make sure to keep your core tight and maintain proper alignment throughout.

- Inhale as you lower your chest and exhale as you push back up.

5. Progress to Kneeling Push-Ups
- Start by kneeling on the floor with your knees about hip-width apart. Place your hands on the floor, slightly wider than shoulder-width apart, with your fingers spread for better support.

- If you struggle with knee pain, place a pillow under your knees for added support.

- Keep your body in a straight line from your head to your knees. Engage your core to prevent your hips from sagging or arching.

- Bend your elbows and lower your chest toward the chair in a controlled manner. Keep your elbows at a 45-degree angle from your body, not flaring out too wide. Press through your palms to straighten your arms, lifting your chest back up to the starting position. Make sure to keep your core tight and maintain proper alignment throughout.

- Inhale as you lower your chest and exhale as you push back up.

7. Full Push-Up
- Slowly bend your elbows and lower your chest towards the floor, keeping your elbows at a 45-degree angle to your body. Make sure your body remains straight throughout the movement, with your core tight and hips in line with your

shoulders and feet.

- Press through your palms and push your body back up to the starting position, fully extending your arms. Keep your core engaged and avoid letting your hips sag.

- Inhale as you lower your chest and exhale as you push back up.

Benefits of These Progressions

The progressions build upper body strength, particularly targeting the chest, shoulders, while also improving shoulder stability and promoting proper alignment during pushing movements. It engages the core and stabilizing muscles, supporting overall posture and balance. Additionally, this exercise enhances endurance and control, which translates into better performance of functional daily tasks, making it a valuable addition to any fitness routine.

** Progression for Calf Raises **

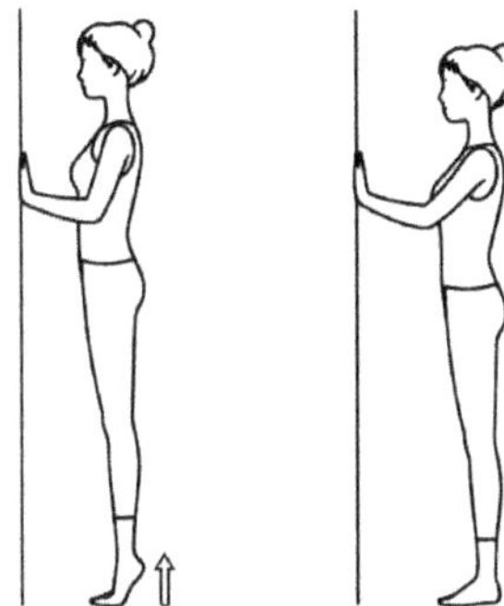

The standing calf raise builds on the seated version by introducing a balance challenge, further strengthening the lower body and improving ankle mobility. It also engages the muscles of the feet and lower legs, promoting better posture and safer movement during daily activities.

Progression Steps

1. Seated Calf Raises (Bodyweight)
   - Build endurance and familiarize yourself with the movement. Sit with your feet flat on the ground, knees bent at 90 degrees, and perform calf raises by lifting your heels as high as possible.

   - Start with bodyweight only and focus on a **full range of motion** and **controlled tempo** (2 seconds up, 2 seconds down).

2. Seated Calf Raises (Weighted)
   - Gradually increase resistance to build strength. Place a weight (barbell, dumbbell, or something that can add some weight evenly) across your knees.

   - Gradually increase the weight while maintaining proper form. Add a **pause at the top** (1-2 seconds) to maximize contraction.

3. Tempo-Controlled Seated Calf Raises
   - Improve control and muscle endurance. Perform each repetition with a **3-4 second eccentric phase** (slow the movement on the lowering phase) and a 1-second pause at the bottom.

- Gradually increase the duration of the eccentric phase (up to 5 seconds).

4. Single-Leg Seated Calf Raises

- Correct imbalances and increase stability by performing the exercise with one foot at a time, keeping the other foot elevated.

- Start with bodyweight, then add light resistance as you progress.

5. Elevated Seated Calf Raises

- Increase range of motion for a deeper stretch and fuller contraction by placing your feet on an elevated surface (e.g., a step or platform) while performing seated calf raises and progress as indicated in Step 1-5 with an elevation.

- Perform slow, controlled movements to maximize stretch at the bottom.

6. Standing Calf Raise Progression

- Once you've built a solid foundation with seated calf raises, transition to standing variations following the same process as steps 1-6 in a standing position.

- Perform slow, controlled movements to maximize stretch at the bottom and contract the core to keep a perfect alignment and void injuries.

Using Resistance Bands for Balance

Resistance bands are versatile tools that have found their place in many fitness routines and are a tool that my husband and I use in our online classes. They offer a unique way to enhance balance training by providing variable resistance, which helps build muscle strength and improve stability through controlled movements. This concept might seem complex, but it's quite straightforward. When you stretch a resistance band, it creates tension that your muscles must work against. This resistance is what helps build strength. It's like having a portable gym in your hands, ready to assist you in your balance training wherever you are. The beauty of resistance bands lies in their simplicity and effectiveness, making them ideal for those looking to improve their balance without investing in heavy equipment.

When using resistance bands, safety and correct usage are paramount. Before each session, inspect your bands for wear and tear. Bands can deteriorate over time, and using a damaged band can lead to injury. Ensure there are no cracks or weak spots. If you notice any damage, it's time to replace the band. Properly securing the band during exercises is also crucial. If the band slips, it can snap back, causing injury. I would suggest starting with a band that offers light resistance, especially if you're new to these exercises. As you become more confident, you can progress to bands with higher resistance, which will further challenge your muscles and improve your balance.

This gradual increase in resistance continues to challenge your muscles, promoting further strength gains. Additionally, you can incorporate more complex movements to keep your routine engaging and effective. For example, try combining arm movements with your leg lifts or incorporating balance challenges, like standing on one foot while using the band. These variations not only make your workouts more interesting but also enhance your overall balance and coordination.

Resistance bands offer a dynamic and adaptable way to enhance your balance training. They are compact, lightweight, and versatile, making them a valuable addition to any fitness routine. Whether you're at home, in the park, or even travelling, these bands provide an effective means to strengthen your muscles and improve your stability. As you explore the possibilities with resistance bands, remember to focus on safety, proper form, and progression. Embrace the challenge, and enjoy the benefits that come with enhanced strength and balance.

Combining Exercises for Maximum Benefit

Combining exercises into a cohesive routine can transform a standard workout into something truly beneficial. By integrating different exercises, you engage multiple muscle groups simultaneously, which enhances both cardiovascular and muscular endurance. This approach not only saves time but also maximizes the effectiveness of each session.

Circuit training is often an approach I like to use when the client becomes stronger and is ready for a new challenge. It entails moving from one exercise to the next with minimal rest. This keeps your heart rate elevated and challenges various muscles in novel ways. Imagine performing a series of balance exercises, followed by strength training and then coordination drills. Each component complements the others, creating a well-rounded workout that addresses all aspects of fitness. Supersetting is another effective strategy. By pairing complementary exercises, like squats followed by lunges, you maintain intensity while targeting different muscle groups. This method keeps your body engaged and reduces downtime, making the most of your workout.

The diversity of combined exercises not only enhances physical benefits but also keeps workouts interesting and challenging. This variety helps prevent boredom, a common barrier to maintaining a regular exercise routine. When you incorporate different movements and techniques, each session feels fresh and engaging, which can boost motivation. Moreover, varied exercises prevent plateaus by continuously challenging the body in different ways. When the body adapts to a routine, progress can stall. By mixing exercises, you encourage continuous improvement, keeping your fitness journey dynamic and rewarding. This adaptability is crucial, especially as you age because it allows you to tailor your workouts to your changing needs and capabilities.

Creating a personalized exercise routine involves balancing intensity with recovery. It's important to listen to your body and adjust your routine based on how you feel. For those just starting, begin with lower-intensity exercises and gradually increase the difficulty as your fitness improves. Tailoring exercises to your fitness level ensures that you're challenging yourself without risking injury. Consider incorporating rest days to allow your body to recover and adapt. These days, they can be used for active recovery activities like walking or gentle stretching, which aid in muscle repair and prevent burnout. Remember, the goal is to maintain a sustainable routine that supports long-term health and well-being.

When designing custom exercise combinations, align them with your individual goals. If your aim is to improve balance, include exercises that challenge your stability and coordination. For those focusing on strength, prioritize resistance and weight-bearing exercises. It's also beneficial to set specific, measurable goals to track your progress. This could be increasing the number of repetitions or the duration of each exercise. Having clear objectives not only provides direction but also fosters a sense of accomplishment as you achieve them. Tracking your progress through a journal or app can offer insights into what works best for you, enabling you to fine-tune your routine over time.

Incorporating these elements into your fitness routine requires commitment and creativity, but the rewards are well worth the effort. By combining exercises, you optimize your workout, making it more efficient and effective. This approach supports a balanced development of strength, endurance, and flexibility, which are essential for maintaining independence and quality of life. The beauty of this method lies in its adaptability; you can modify your routine to suit your changing needs and preferences. Whether you're exercising at home, in a gym, or even outdoors, combining exercises offers a versatile and engaging way to improve your fitness.

CONCLUSION

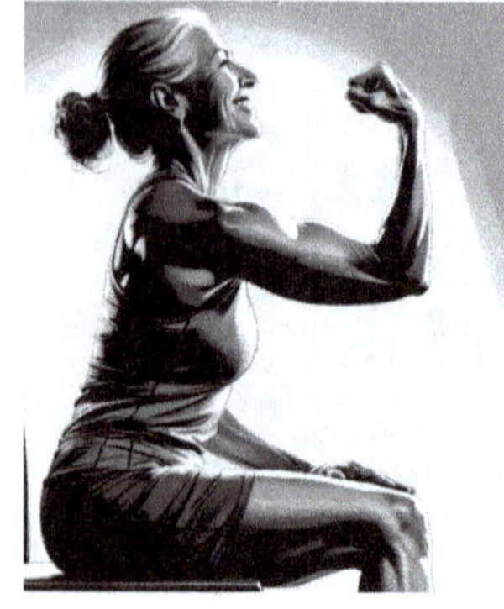

As you reach this final chapter, let's revisit the journey we've embarked on together. This book has been your guide to enhancing strength, balance and coordination, vital components for maintaining independence and confidence in your daily life. We've explored exercises designed to be safe and accessible, gradually increasing in complexity to accommodate all fitness levels. These workouts aim to empower you to move with assurance, reducing the risk of falls and giving you the freedom to engage fully in the activities you love.

Balance and coordination are not just skills; they are lifelines. They allow you to navigate your surroundings with ease, perform daily tasks with confidence, and participate fully in social activities. By focusing on these areas, you protect yourself from the potential hazards of falls, one of the leading causes of injury among seniors. As you continue to practice these exercises, you'll find that your confidence grows, along with your ability to enjoy each day to the fullest.

Reflecting on my journey, I am reminded of the inspiration behind this book—my grandmother. Her resilience and determination to maintain her independence sparked my passion for senior fitness. My own path from gymnast to personal trainer was not without challenges. I've faced injuries and health issues, but these experiences have only fueled my commitment to helping others. This book is a testament to the power of perseverance and the belief that it's never too late to become a better version of yourself.

Throughout this book, you've learned the importance of consistency in exercise. Regular practice is key to maintaining the progress you've made. We've also emphasized a holistic approach, incorporating mindfulness and nutrition to support overall well-being. Setting realistic goals is crucial; they provide direction and motivation, helping you to measure your achievements and set new challenges. While this book serves as a foundation, the journey doesn't end here. The exercises and practices you've learned are tools for a lifetime. By integrating them into your daily routine, you will continue to build strength, improve balance, and enhance your quality of life. Share your progress with family and friends; let them be your cheerleaders and motivators. Seek out community support, whether it be a local fitness group or an online community, to stay inspired and accountable.

I encourage you to use the practical resources that have been sprinkled in this book, as they have been created to support you on this journey. Learning from past experience I realize how helpful these tools can be in attaining your fitness goals. You will find a dedicated section for establishing your SMART goals that will guide your progress. Additionally, you'll find a personalized exercise log and a comprehensive evaluation in the Appendix, designed to capture your initial fitness level and monitor your advancements at each retest interval. This tailored approach ensures you can visibly track your successes and areas for improvement. Moreover, I've compiled a selection of exercises accompanied by detailed diagrams and explanations to make sure you are able to reproduce the movements in their proper form and with ease. This collection allows you to customize your workout regimen based on your current mobility level and how you feel on any given day, ensuring a personalized and adaptable fitness journey.

Finally, I want to express my deepest gratitude for taking this journey with me. Your dedication to improving your health is inspiring. Celebrate your achievements, no matter how small. Embrace the changes you have made and continue to strive for a healthier, more independent lifestyle. As you continue on this path, keep in mind this quote: *"Age is no barrier. It's a limitation you put on your mind."* Let this sentiment guide you, reminding you that the power to change and grow is always within your reach. Thank you for allowing me to be part of your journey, and here's to a future filled with health, happiness, and endless possibilities.

APPENDIX

Home Assessment – Seated

Date:_______________

1. Seated Leg Extension

- Sit in a sturdy chair or wheelchair with feet flat on the ground.

- Extend one leg out straight, hold for a moment, and then lower it back down.

- Repeat with the other leg.

- Complete as many times as possible in 30 seconds.

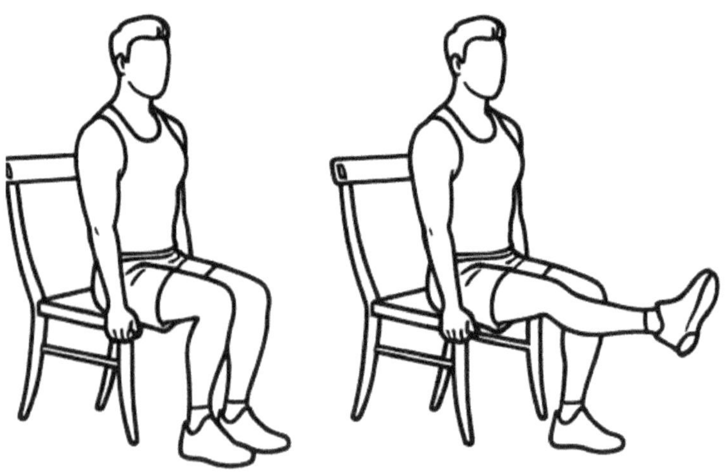

RESULT____________

2. Seated Balance

- Sit in a chair with feet flat on the ground.

- Lift one foot off the ground and hold for as long as possible without support.

- Measure the time the foot is held off the ground for each leg.

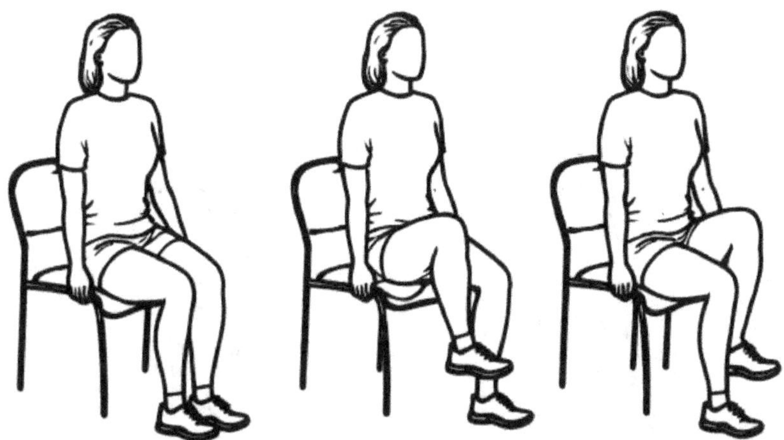

RESULT__________

3. Seated Torso Rotation Test

- Sit upright in a chair

- Cross arms over the chest and rotate the torso to the right and then to the left as far as possible.

- Measure the distance of rotation or how far they can turn without straining.

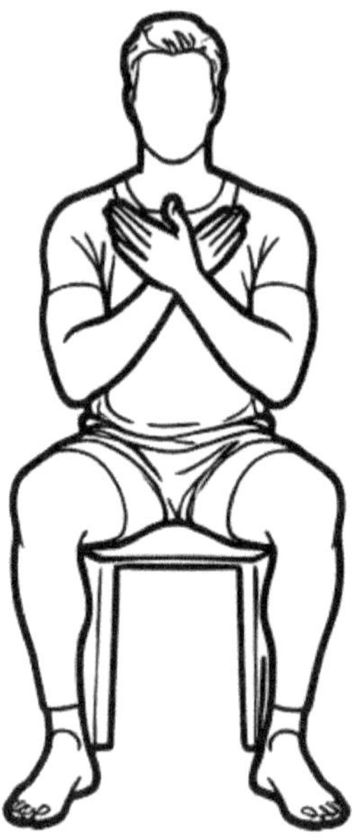 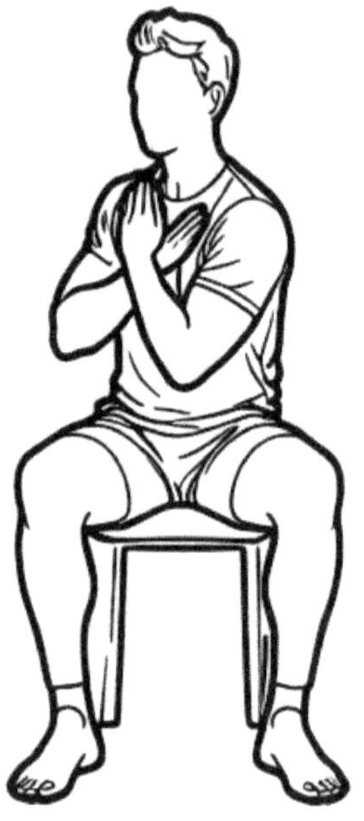

RESULT__________

4. Hand Coordination Test

- Place small objects (e.g., marbles or balls) on a table within reach.

- Attempt to pick them up and place them into a container.

- Count the number of objects transferred within 30 seconds

RESULT__________

5. Breathing Exercises

- Sit comfortably and take deep breaths, inhaling through the nose and exhaling through the mouth.

- Hold each breath for a few seconds before exhaling.

- Note any difficulty with deep breathing and how relaxing you find the exercise.

RESULT______

6. Seated Heel Toe Tap Test

- While seated, alternate tapping the heel and toe of each foot on the floor.

- Count the number of successful taps in 30 seconds

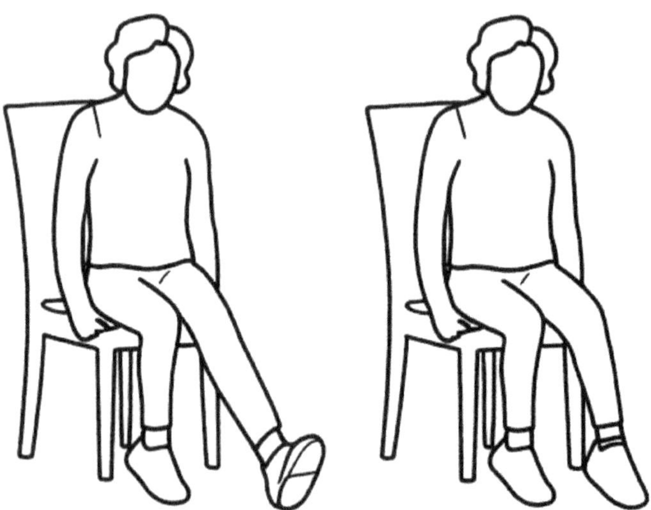

RESULT__________

Home Assessment – Standing

Date:_____________

1. Chair Stand Test

- Start seated in a chair with arms crossed over the chest or in a prayer position.

- Stand up completely and sit back down as many times as possible in 30 seconds.

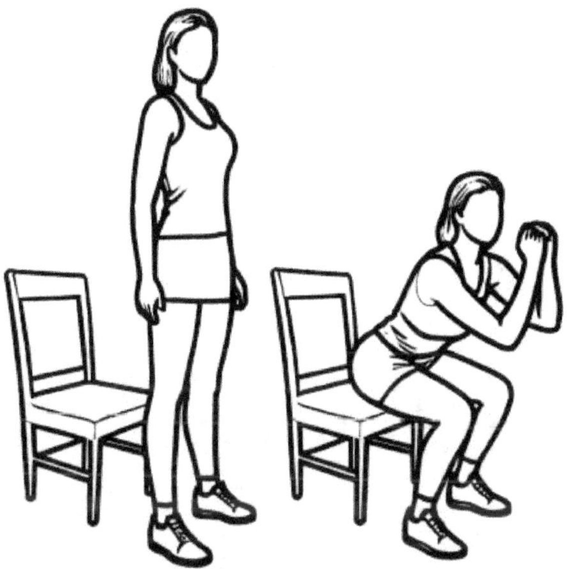

RESULT___________

2. Timed Standing Balance Test (Single Leg Stand)

- Stand on one leg for as long as possible without support.

- Switch legs and repeat. Measure the time on each leg.

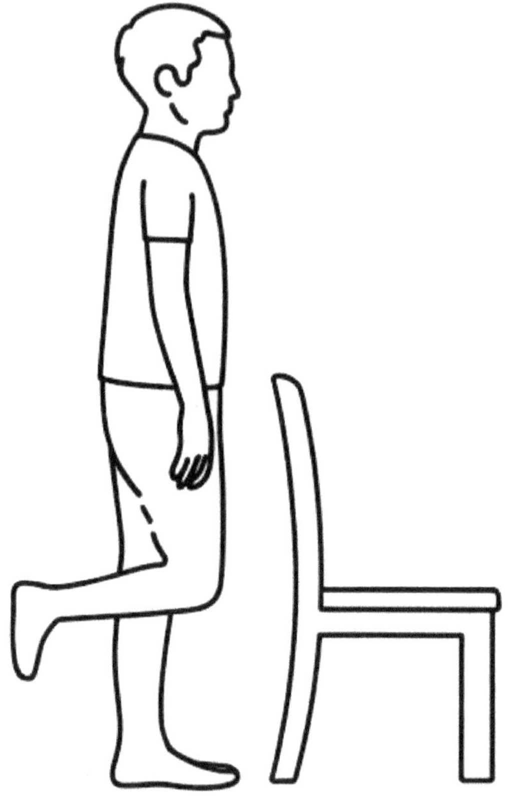

RESULT___________

3. Timed Heel to toe Balance Test

- Place one foot directly in front of the other, with the heel of the front foot touching the toes of the back foot (heel-to-toe position).

- Measure how long you can hold that position standing without losing balance.

- Be sure to stay near a counter top for support.

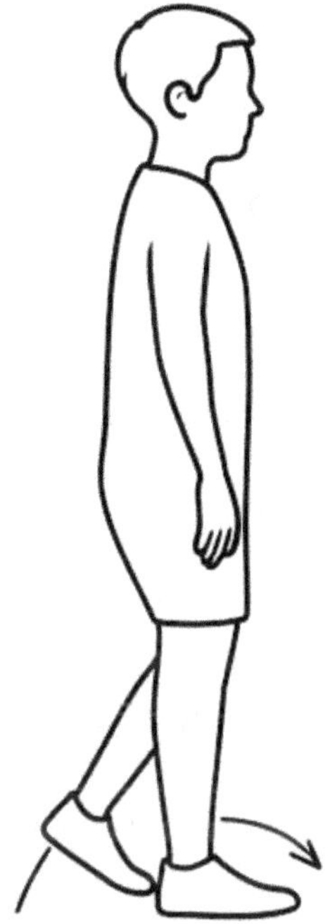
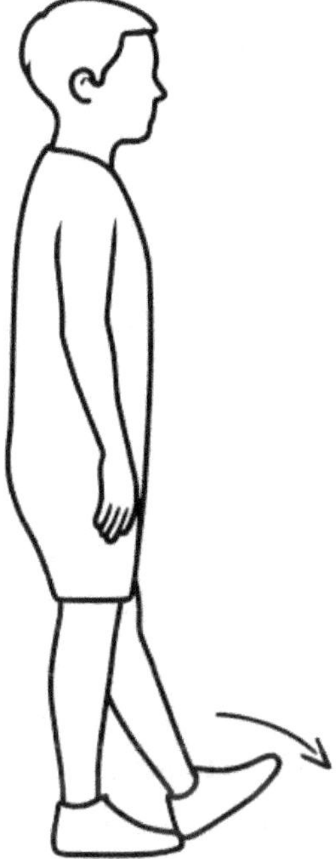

RESULT__________

4. Timed Up and Go (TUG) Test

- Start seated in a chair.

- Stand up, walk 10 feet (3 meters), turn around, walk back, and sit down.

- Measure the time taken to complete the task.

RESULT_________

5. Step Test

- Use a low step (6-8 inches).

- Step up and down at a steady pace for 3 minutes.

- Measure heart rate immediately after completing the test.

  - **How to Measure Your Heart Rate Manually**

    i. **Find a Pulse Point**
    You can feel your pulse at spots where an artery is close to the surface of your skin. The two easiest locations are:

    ii. **Wrist (Radial Pulse):** Place two fingers (index and middle) on the underside of your wrist, just below the base of your thumb.

    iii. **Neck (Carotid Pulse):** Place two fingers gently on the side of your neck, just below your jawbone.

    iv. **Count the Beats**

    - Once you feel your pulse, use a watch, clock, or timer.

    - Count the number of beats you feel in **30 seconds**.

    - Multiply that number by **2** to calculate your beats per minute (BPM).

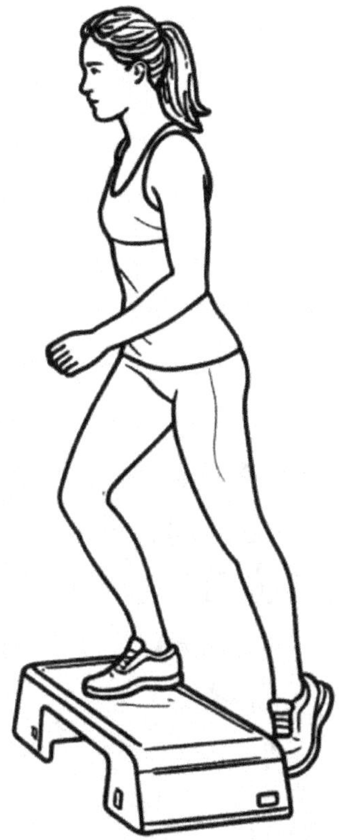

RESULT___________

6. Wall Angel Test

- Stand with the back against a wall, feet about 6 inches away from the wall.

- Raise arms to form a "W" shape, keeping the back, arms, and head in contact
  with the wall.
  Slowly slide arms up to form a "Y" shape and back down to "W."

- Observe if you can maintain contact with the wall throughout the movement.

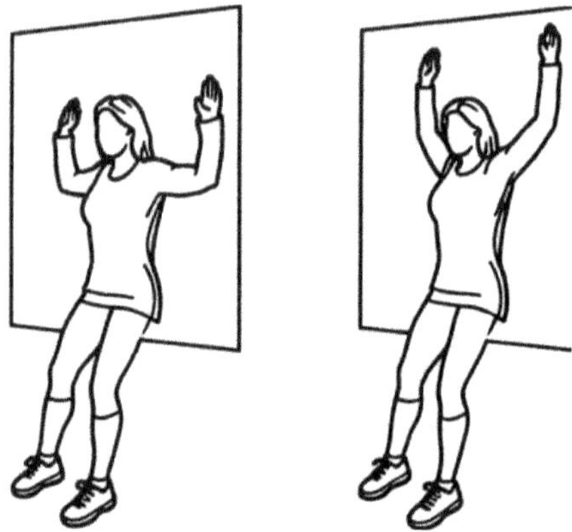

RESULT_____________

REFERENCES

- Healthline. (2023, March 13). *Balance exercises for seniors: 11 moves to try.* Healthline. https://www.healthline.com/health/exercise-fitness/balance-exercises-for-seniors

- Centers for Disease Control and Prevention. (2024, May 16). *About older adult fall prevention.* U.S. Department of Health and Human Services. https://www.cdc.gov/falls/about/index.html

- Centers for Disease Control and Prevention (CDC). (2024, June 4). *About older adult fall prevention.* CDC. https://www.cdc.gov/falls/about/index.html

- Wu, Y., et al. (2021). Age-related vestibular loss and associated deficits. *Journal of Vestibular Research*, 31(2), 107-116. https://doi.org/10.3233/VES-200912

- Mayo Clinic. (2023). *Fall prevention: Simple tips to prevent falls.* Mayo Clinic. https://www.mayoclinic.org/healthy-lifestyle/healthy-aging/in-depth/fall-prevention/art-20047358

- Lifeline. (n.d.). 14 exercises for seniors to improve strength and balance. Lifeline. https://www.lifeline.ca/en/resources/14-exercises-for-seniors-to-improve-strength-and-balance/

- Health Education Partners. (n.d.). Exercise for healthy aging: SMART goal & FITT principle. Health Education Partners. https://www.healthedpartners.org/ceu/pa-healthyaging/Create_Healthy_Aging_Exercise_Program.pdf

- Mayo Clinic. (2019, October 9). *Fall prevention: Simple tips to prevent falls.* Mayo Clinic. https://www.mayoclinic.org/healthy-lifestyle/healthy-aging/in

-depth/fall-prevention/art-20047358□97†source□□98†source□.

- SilverSneakers. (2023, May 29). *5 warm-up exercises for seniors: Tips from the experts*. SilverSneakers. https://www.silversneakers.com/blog/warm-up-exerci se/□89†source□□90†source□.

- SilverSneakers. (2023, May 29). *6 best balance exercises for seniors to improve stability*. SilverSneakers. https://www.silversneakers.com/blog/balance-exerci ses-seniors/

- Goh, S. (2020).*Musculoskeletal pain in older adults*. National Institutes of Health. https://www.ncbi.nlm.nih.gov/pmc/articles/PMC8034863/

- National Institutes of Health (NIH). (2020). *Effectiveness of Tai Chi for health promotion of older adults*. NIH. https://www.ncbi.nlm.nih.gov/pmc/articles/ PMC9644143/

- American Council on Exercise (ACE). (2020, February 28). *Chair yoga poses: 7 poses for better balance*. ACE Fitness. https://www.acefitness.org/resources/ev eryone/blog/5478/chair-yoga-poses-7-poses-for-better-balance/

- Conservatory Senior Living. (n.d.). *How to assess seniors' fitness progress*. Conservatory Senior Living. https://www.conservatoryseniorliving.com/senior-liv ing-blog/how-to-assess-seniors-fitness-progress/

- National Institutes of Health (NIH). (2016, November 1). *Mindfulness-based interventions for older adults*. NIH. https://www.ncbi.nlm.nih.gov/pmc/arti cles/PMC4868399/

- Amica. (2024, January 2). *Seniors, use mindful breathing to manage stress or anxiety*. Amica. https://www.amica.ca/conversations/seniors-use-mindful-br eathing-to-manage-stress-or-anxiety

- U.S. Department of Agriculture. (n.d.). *USDA MyPlate nutrition information for older adults*. MyPlate. https://www.myplate.gov/life-stages/older-adults

- Aegis Living. (n.d.). *The importance of staying hydrated for seniors*. Aegis Living. https://www.aegisliving.com/resource-center/the-importance-of-staying

-hydrated/

- Mayo Clinic. (2023, February 17). *Exercising with arthritis: Improve your joint pain and stiffness.* Mayo Clinic. https://www.mayoclinic.org/diseases-conditions/arthritis/in-depth/arthritis/art-20047971

- MoreLife Health. (2024, April 10). *Flexibility exercises for seniors: A comprehensive guide.* MoreLife Health https://morelifehealth.com/articles/regaining-flexibility-guide

- Harvard Health. (2023, December 3). *Don't be the fall guy.* Harvard Health Publishing. https://www.health.harvard.edu/staying-healthy/dont-be-the-fall-guy

- ParentGiving. (2024, June 15). *Exercise for seniors with limited mobility.* ParentGiving. https://www.parentgiving.com/blogs/patient-daily-living/exercise-for-seniors-with-limited-mobility

- Senior Lifestyle. (n.d.). *How group exercise programs benefit seniors.* https://www.seniorlifestyle.com/resources/blog/benefits-of-group-fitness-classes/

- Cozy Chris. (n.d.). *34 senior fitness quotes for inspiration.* https://cozychris.com/senior-fitness-quotes/

- Adamson, W. (n.d.). *Over 50 and hit a training plateau? Here's what to do.* https://www.walteradamson.com/blog/how-to-break-through-exercise-plateaus

- SilverSneakers. (n.d.). *Functional exercises for seniors: Improve balance and stability.* https://www.silversneakers.com/blog/functional-fitness-the-silversneakers-guide/

- Abbey Delray. (n.d.). *Benefits of balance exercises for older adults.* https://www.abbeydelray.com/blog/benefits-of-balance-exercises-for-older-adults/

- Seniors.com.au. (n.d.). *Exercising when you're over 50: Best practices and tips.* https://www.seniors.com.au/funeral-insurance/discover/exercising-over-50

- Synctuition. (n.d.). *Why making time for evening relaxation is important.* https://synctuition.com/blog/why-making-time-for-evening-relaxation

-is-important-and-how-to-do-it/

- National Center for Biotechnology Information (NCBI). (n.d.). *Effect of chair yoga therapy on functional fitness.* PMC. https://www.ncbi.nlm.nih.gov/pmc/articles/PMC10094373/

- SilverSneakers. (n.d.). *The total-body resistance band workout.* https://www.silversneakers.com/blog/total-body-resistance-band-workout-older-adults/

- National Center for Biotechnology Information (NCBI). (n.d.). *Effects of combined balance and strength training on health outcomes.* PMC. https://www.ncbi.nlm.nih.gov/pmc/articles/PMC7786296/

- CloSler. (n.d.). *Mindful movement.* https://closler.org/lifelong-learning-in-clinical-excellence/mindful-movement

- TheYCollection. (n.d.). *20+ best exercises to improve gut health.* https://theycollection.com/blogs/biohub/exercise-for-gut-health

- Sleepie.ai. (n.d.). *How much deep sleep should you get every night?.* https://sleepie.ai/how-much-deep-sleep-should-you-get-every-night/

- MAGMA Fitness. (n.d.). *How to use resistance bands for maximum fitness benefits.* https://magmafitness.com/blogs/magma-blog/how-to-use-resistance-bands-for-maximum-fitness-benefits

- Live Positively. (n.d.). *6 easy ways to boost your balance.* https://livepositively.com/6-easy-ways-to-boost-your-balance/